KETO BEGINNERS GUIDE
FOR WOMEN OVER 50

The Ultimate Ketogenic Diet Cookbook for Seniors with Low Carb Recipes and DIY Face Masks For Anti-Aging Effect

Kathrin Narrell

COPYRIGHT © 2020 BY KATHRIN NARRELL

ALL RIGHTS RESERVED.

No part of this book may be reproduced in any form or by any electronic or mechanical means, except in the case of a brief quotation embodied in articles or reviews, without written permission from its publisher.

DISCLAIMER

The recipes and information in this book are provided for educational purposes only. Please always consult a licensed professional before making changes to your lifestyle or diet. The author and publisher shall have neither liability nor responsibility to anyone with respect to any loss or damage caused or alleged to be caused directly or indirectly by the information contained in this book. All trademarks and brands within this book are for clarifying purposes only and are owned by the owners themselves, not affiliated with this document.

Images from shutterstock.com

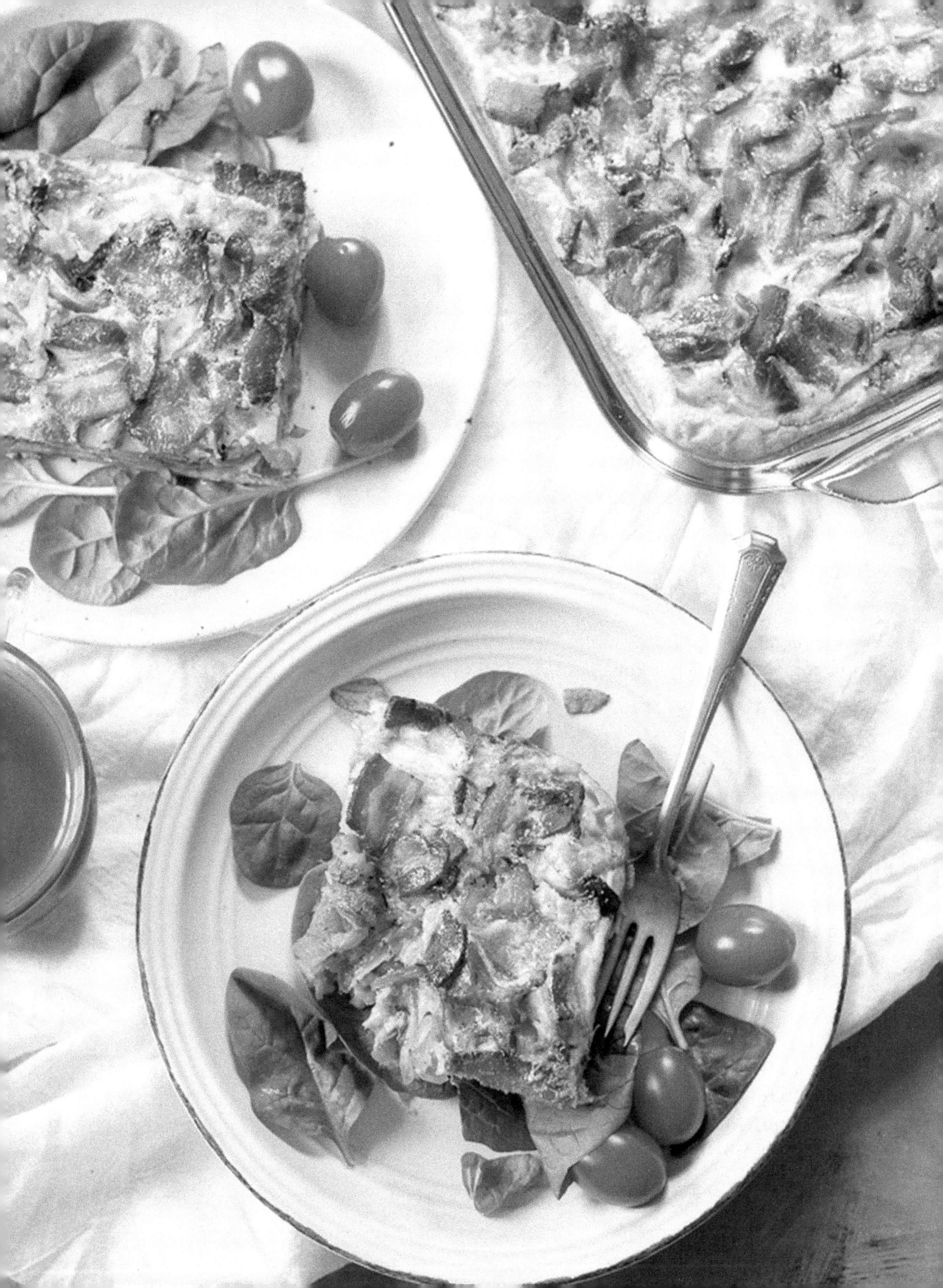

CONTENTS

INTRODUCTION 7
CHAPTER 1. KETO OVERVIEW 8
    11 Keto foods... 8
    Best Fruits on Keto 9
    Best Vegetbles on Keto.. 10
    Best Nuts on Keto 11
    Best Snacks on Keto 11
    Best Dairy on Keto 12
    Best Flour on Keto 13
    Best Alcohol on Keto 13
    Best Sweeteners on Keto 14
    What is Ketosis? 14
    Beauty tips from Keto Products 15
CHAPTER 2. EGG MASKS 16
    Softening Mask 16
    Antiaging Mask 16
    Nourishing Mask 16
    Tonic Mask 16
    Cleansing Mask 17
    Antiaging Mask for Dry Skin 17
CHAPTER 3. AVOCADO MASKS 18
    Avocado Mask for Dry Skin 18
    Avocado Mask for Oily Skin 18
    Avocado Mask for Flaky Skin 18
CHAPTER 4. RECIPES 19
EGG RECIPES 19
    Omelet in a Cup 19
    Goat Cheese Frittata 20
    Squash Frittata 21
    Scotch Quail Eggs 22
    Mediterranean Delived Eggs 23
    Egg Paste 24
    Mushrooms stuffed with Eggs 25
    Broccoli Omelet 26
    Eggs Florentine 27
    Egg and Shrimp Salad 28
BACON RECIPES 29
    Bacon and Egg Fat Bombs 29

Fried BAcon and Cabbage 30
Bacon Wrapped Chicken 31
Bacon Wrapped Mozzarella 32
Bacon Ties 33
Romaine Salad 34
Warm Bacon and Arugula Salad 35
BAcon Salad with Walnuts 36
Bacon and Pear Salad 37
No Bread BTL 38

AVOCADO RECIPES 39

Avocado and Shrimp Salad 39
Avocado and Cucumber Salad 40
Avocado Salsa 41
Avocado Salad 42
Avocado Spring Rolls 43
Avocado Bowl 44
Avocado Casserole 45
Avocado Feta Dip 46
Prosciutto-Wrapped Avocado 47
Cucumber Rolls with Avocado 48
Avocado and Tuna Brown Rice 49
Avocado Ice Cream 50
Avocado Bars 51

GREEN VEGETABLES RECIPES 52

Cabbage Patties 52
Cabbage and Egg Salad 53
Kale Salad 54
Green Eastern Salad 55
Chicken Fillets Baked with Broccoli 56
Broccoli and Mushroom Quiche title 57
Broccoli in Orange Sauce 58
Spinach with Tomatoes 59
Spinach Salad with Tuna 60
spinach Rolls 61
Mozzarella Spinach 62
Lettuce Wraps 63

BEVERAGES 64

Lavender Glass 64
Ginger Cooler 65
Apple Peel Tea 66
Cilanro Brew 67

Chicory Coffee 68
Turmeric Power 69
Cold Chocolate 70
Vodka Mojito 71
Tom Collins 72
Wasabi Margarita 73

CONCLUSION 74
RECIPE INDEX 75
CONVERSION TABLES 76

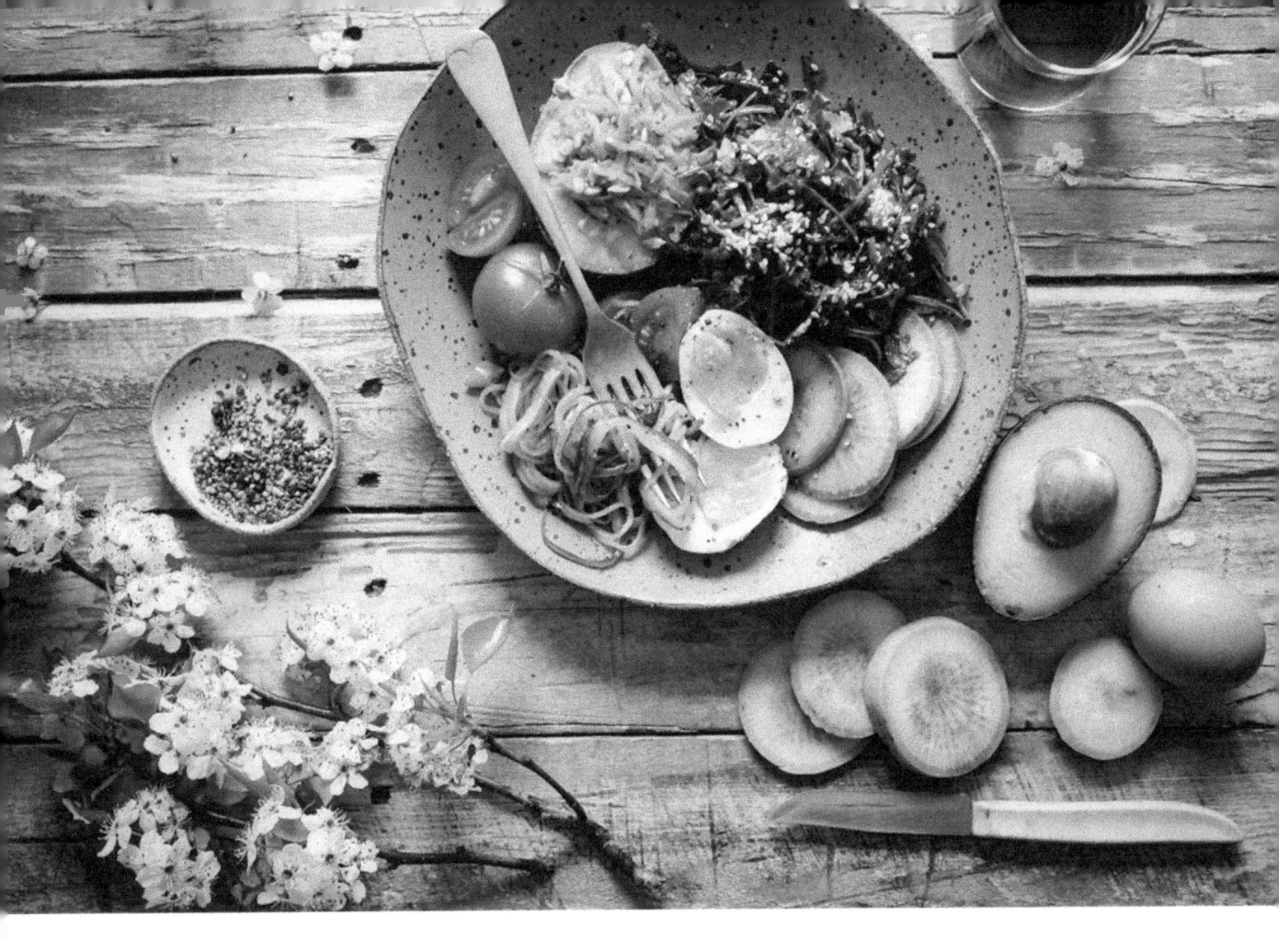

INTRODUCTION

Don't blame the butter for what the bread did. This is a well-known Keto Diet motto, which actually explains a lot since the diet implies ratcheting down the carbohydrates and getting the most energy from fats. You may be called Captain Bacon, Mrs. Greasy or whatever but switching from carbs to fats does provide more power and health.

Since this book was designed for beginners, the recipes are sorted by top keto ingredients plus the beverages section. The eggs are the number one quality protein source; bacon and avocado are two of the top fat sources on keto, and green vegetables grown above ground are responsible for high level of nutrients. Also, because the cookbook is for newbies, it is full of images and charts rather than dry theory. The Keto Diet is not a zero-carb diet but a low-carb diet. A low-carb diet suggests that you eat fewer carbohydrates and a higher portion of fat.sample

Fat

75% of the day's calories from fat (i.e. avocados)

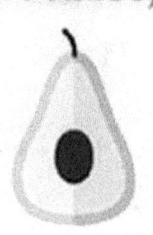

Protein

20% of the day's calories from protein (i.e. fish)

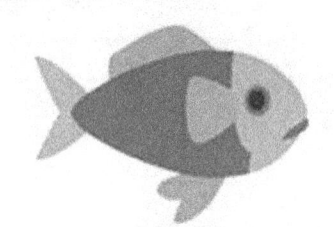

Carbs

5% of the day's calories from carbs (i.e. root veggies)

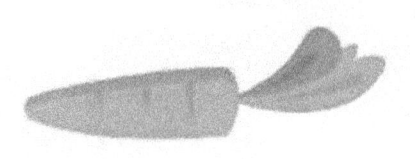

CHAPTER 1. KETO OVERVIEW

11 KETO FOODS

Normal If the great bulk of your kilocalories come from these foods while you are on the Keto Diet, then you will be able to get the most benefits from restricting carbs.

- **Eggs**

As it happens, most of the valuable nutrients in eggs are found in their yolks. One large egg contains less than 1 gram of carbs and fewer than 6 grams of protein, making it the perfect low-carb keto-friendly food.

- **Avocados**

A super product that is second to none. Avocados are packed with nutrients and fatty acids, and are better to consume raw.

- **High-fat dairy**

If you choose to include dairy in your Keto Diet, these should be pastured products from grass-fed cows, butter and, happily, cheese.

- **Meat, poultry, and seafood**

To get the most protein from your meat, it is best to have 100% grass-fed, pasture-raised red meat, pasture-raised poultry and fish that is caught wild like tuna, cod, halibut, salmon, mackerel, snapper, trout, and catfish.

- **Dark chocolate**

You don't really have a free pass to eating cacao in any amount you want, but it does provide us with antioxidants.

- **Olives and olive oil**

Olive oil, apart from low carb and plenty of fat concentration, possesses essential anti-inflammatory properties.

- **Nuts and seeds**

Nuts and seeds will cause no harm, only benefits. See in the charts below what are the best nuts on keto.

- **Berries**

On a Ketogenic Diet we highlight only the following types of berries since their carb levels are relatively low:
blackberries, blueberries, raspberries, strawberries.

- **Cruciferous vegetables**

These are arugula, bok choy, broccoli, Brussels sprouts, cabbage, cauliflower, collard greens.

- **Allium vegetables**

These are onion, garlic, scallion, shallot, leek, and chives.

- **Shirataki noodles**

These are Japanese noodles, which come from the root of an Asian plant. These are a good pasta substitute made up of a viscous fiber.

BEST FRUITS ON KETO

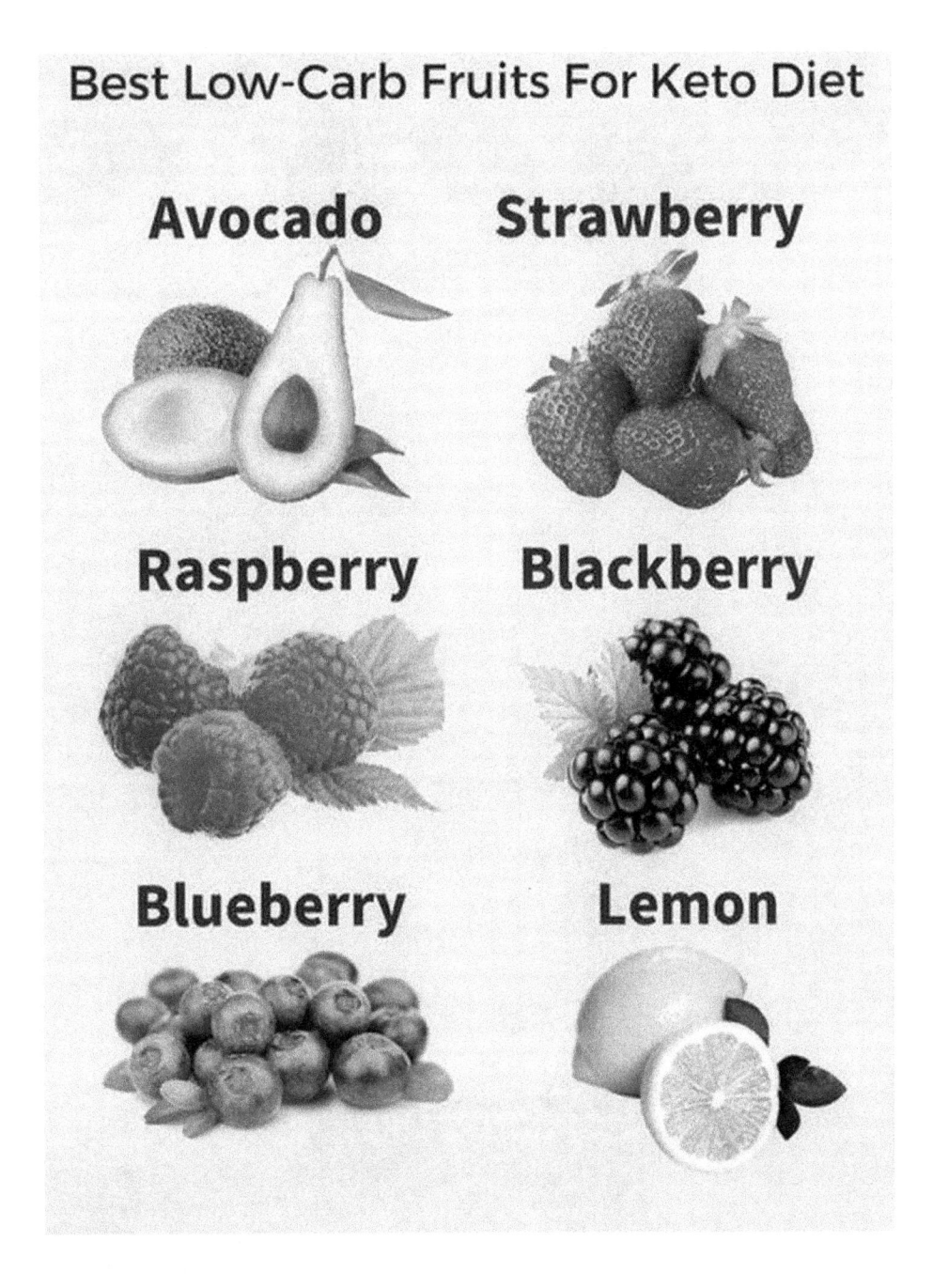

Best Low-Carb Fruits For Keto Diet

- Avocado
- Strawberry
- Raspberry
- Blackberry
- Blueberry
- Lemon

BEST VEGETBLES ON KETO

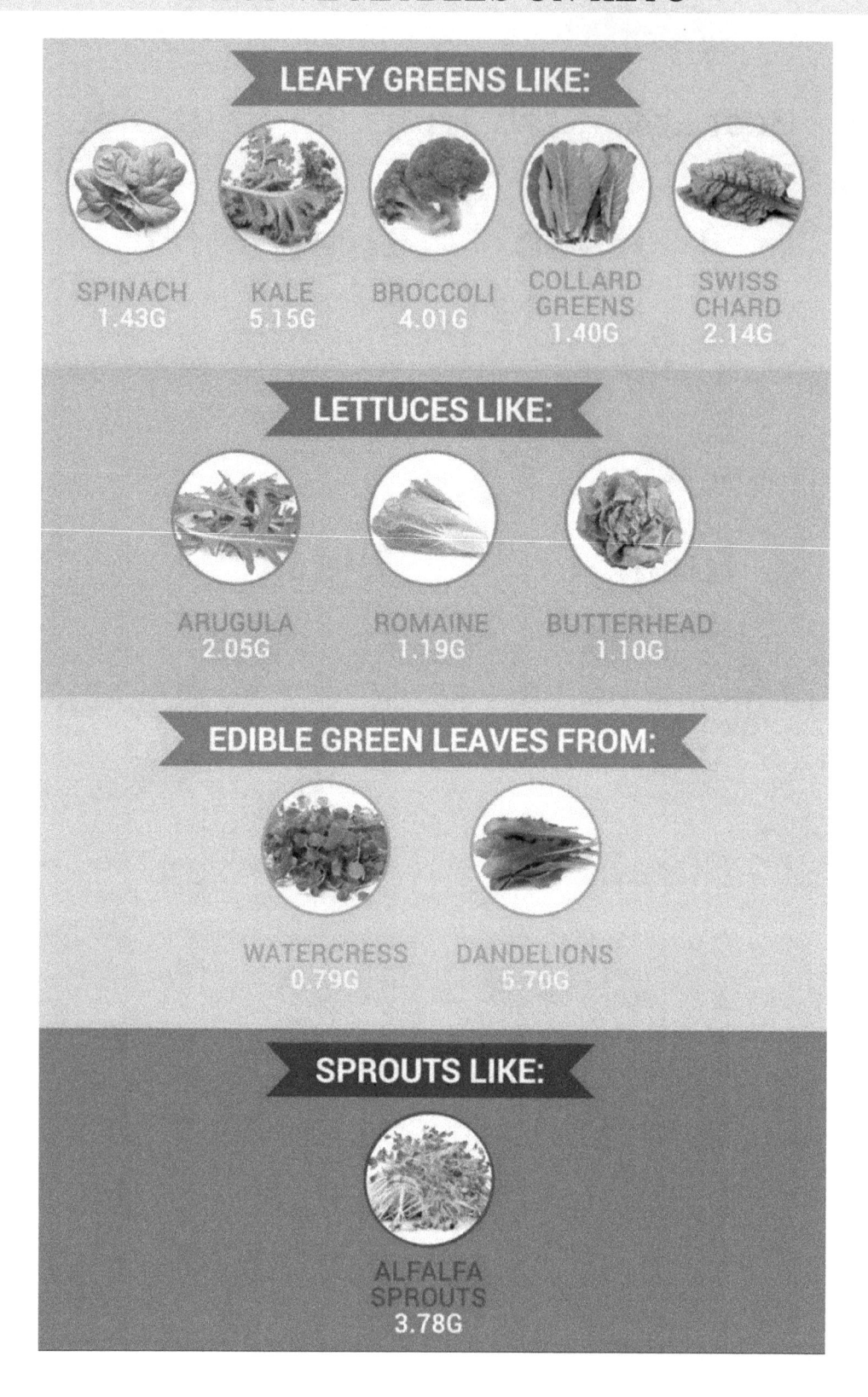

LEAFY GREENS LIKE:
- SPINACH 1.43G
- KALE 5.15G
- BROCCOLI 4.01G
- COLLARD GREENS 1.40G
- SWISS CHARD 2.14G

LETTUCES LIKE:
- ARUGULA 2.05G
- ROMAINE 1.19G
- BUTTERHEAD 1.10G

EDIBLE GREEN LEAVES FROM:
- WATERCRESS 0.79G
- DANDELIONS 5.70G

SPROUTS LIKE:
- ALFALFA SPROUTS 3.78G

Moreover, concentrate on eating green vegetables that grows above the ground like cucumbers, celery, squash, zucchini, asparagus, broccoli, cauliflower, cabbage, eggplants and root vegetables like onion, garlic, radishes. The main point is not eating starchy vegetables, which include potatoes, corn, peas, beans and legumes. It doesn't mean of course you completely cut any other vegetables.

BEST NUTS ON KETO

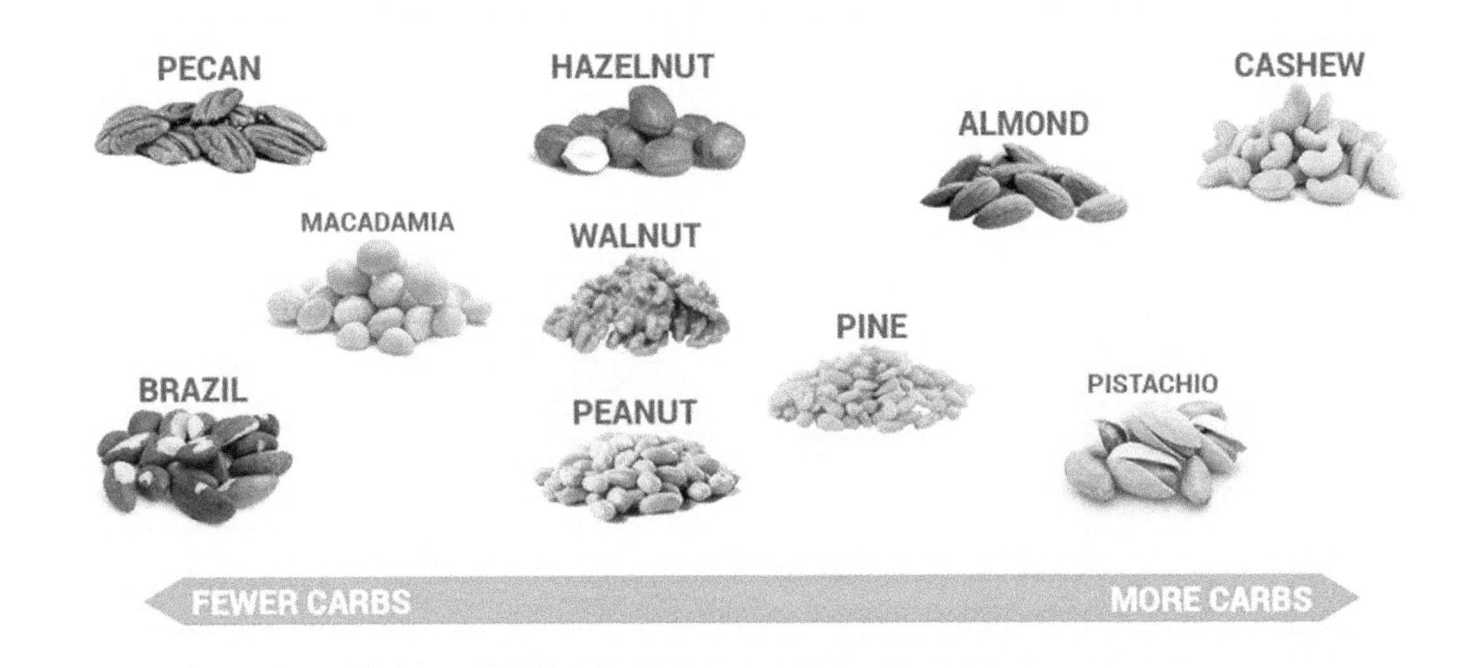

PECAN HAZELNUT ALMOND CASHEW

MACADAMIA WALNUT PINE

BRAZIL PEANUT PISTACHIO

← FEWER CARBS — MORE CARBS →

BEST SNACKS ON KETO

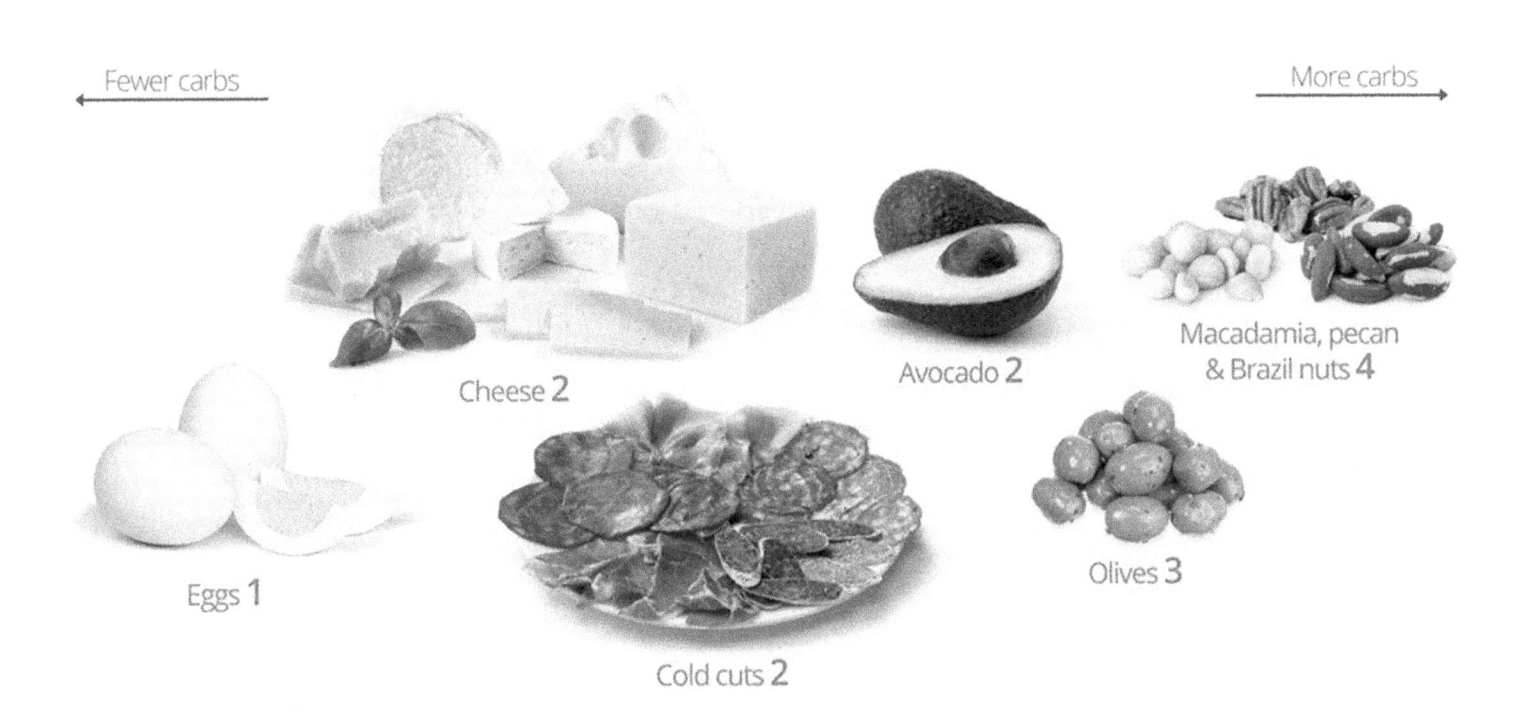

← Fewer carbs   More carbs →

Eggs 1

Cheese 2

Cold cuts 2

Avocado 2

Olives 3

Macadamia, pecan & Brazil nuts 4

BEST DAIRY ON KETO

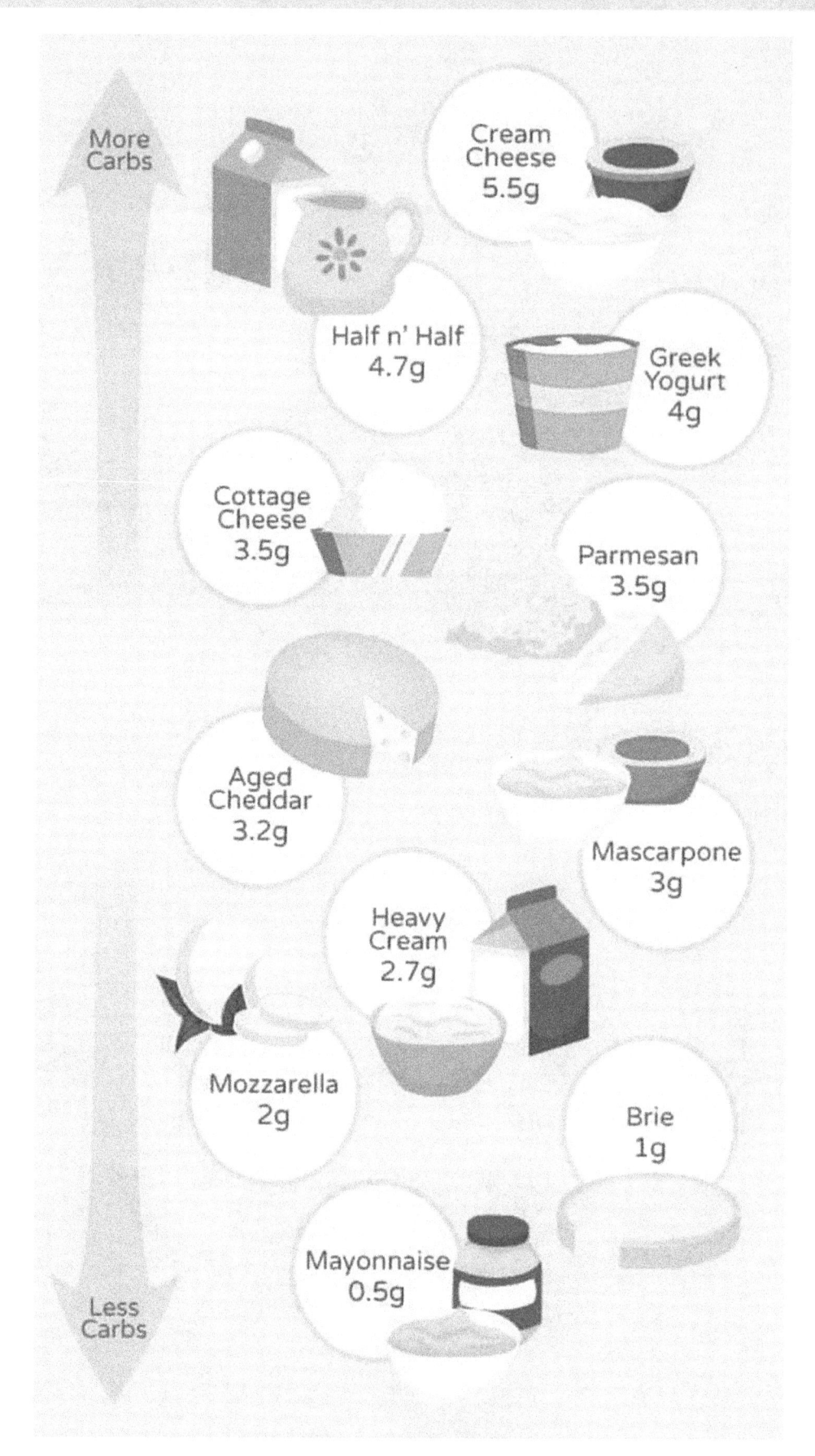

More Carbs ↑

- Cream Cheese 5.5g
- Half n' Half 4.7g
- Greek Yogurt 4g
- Cottage Cheese 3.5g
- Parmesan 3.5g
- Aged Cheddar 3.2g
- Mascarpone 3g
- Heavy Cream 2.7g
- Mozzarella 2g
- Brie 1g
- Mayonnaise 0.5g

Less Carbs ↓

You are allowed to eat full fat dairy products with the exception for milk. Other cheese not mentioned in the chart are also welcomed.

BEST FLOUR ON KETO

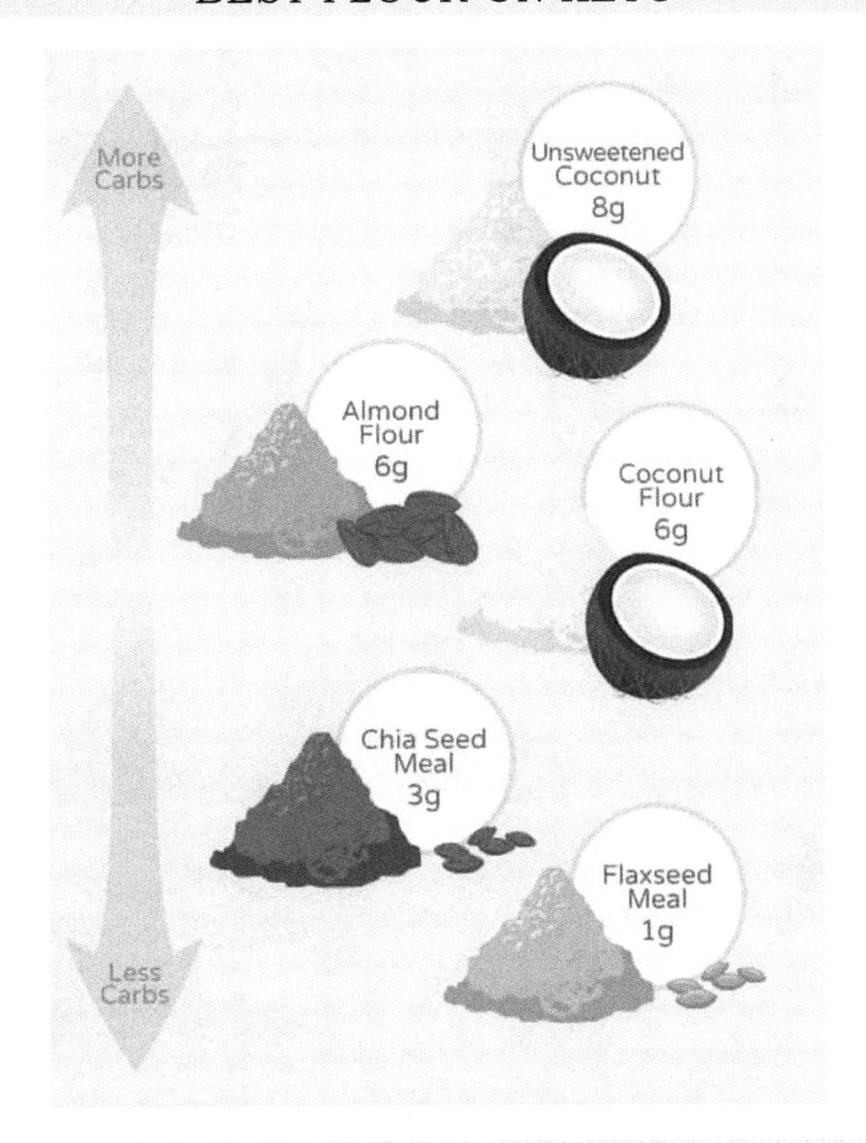

More Carbs ↑

- Unsweetened Coconut 8g
- Almond Flour 6g
- Coconut Flour 6g
- Chia Seed Meal 3g
- Flaxseed Meal 1g

↓ Less Carbs

BEST ALCOHOL ON KETO

Fewer carbs → **More carbs**

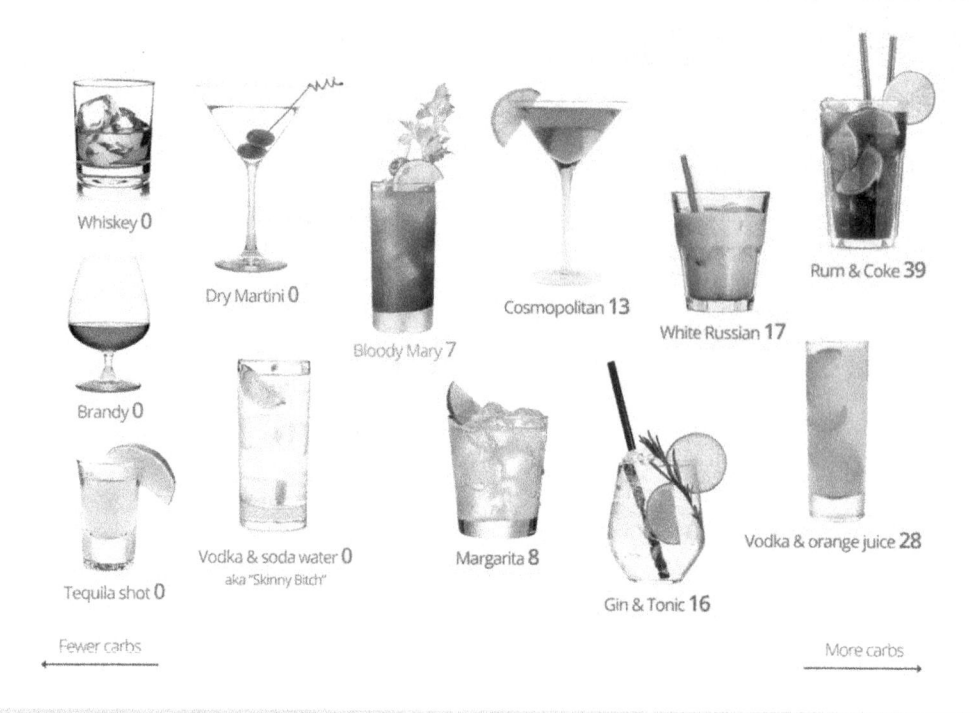

- Whiskey 0
- Dry Martini 0
- Bloody Mary 7
- Cosmopolitan 13
- White Russian 17
- Rum & Coke 39
- Brandy 0
- Vodka & soda water 0 (aka "Skinny Bitch")
- Margarita 8
- Gin & Tonic 16
- Vodka & orange juice 28
- Tequila shot 0

BEST SWEETENERS ON KETO

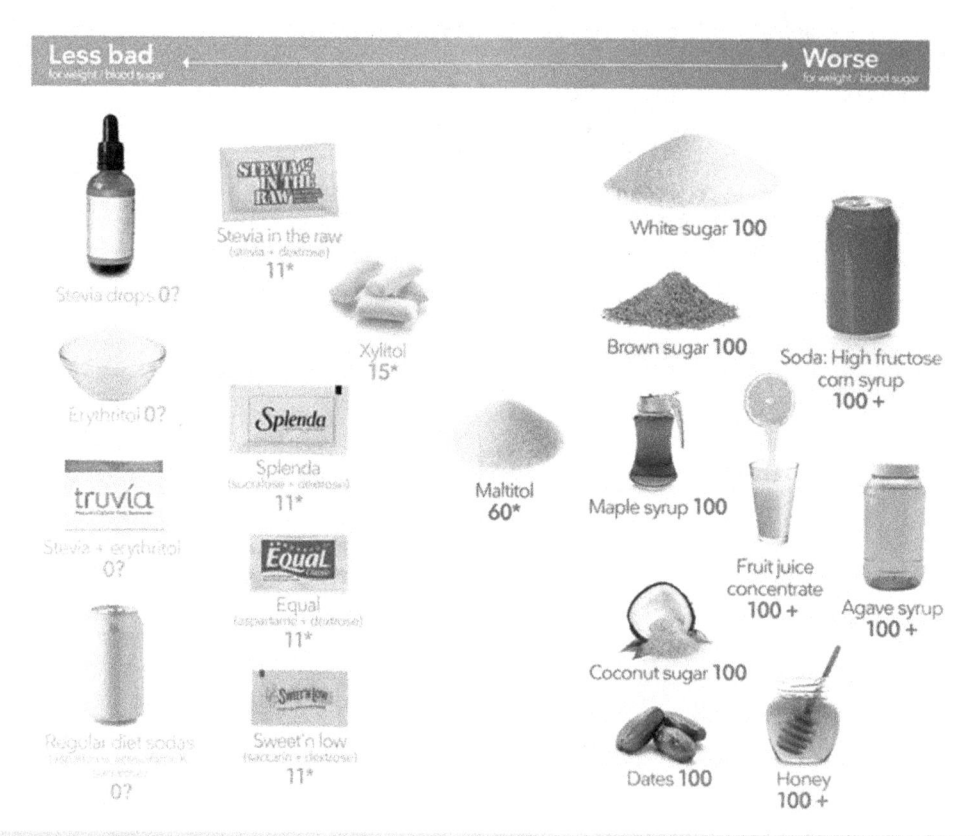

Less bad (for weight / blood sugar) → **Worse** (for weight / blood sugar)

- Stevia drops 0?
- Stevia in the raw (stevia + dextrose) 11*
- Xylitol 15*
- White sugar 100
- Erythritol 0?
- Splenda (sucralose + dextrose) 11*
- Brown sugar 100
- Soda: High fructose corn syrup 100 +
- Truvia (Stevia + erythritol) 0?
- Equal (aspartame + dextrose) 11*
- Maltitol 60*
- Maple syrup 100
- Fruit juice concentrate 100 +
- Agave syrup 100 +
- Regular diet sodas (sucralose, aspartame, acesulfame) 0?
- Sweet'n low (saccharin + dextrose) 11*
- Coconut sugar 100
- Dates 100
- Honey 100 +

WHAT IS KETOSIS?

Ketosis is a state characterized by raised levels of ketone bodies in the body tissues. Ketones are molecules that appear in the blood when fats are broken down for energy. Ketosis occurs when people consume low carb food and the body doesn't have this customary fuel source and starts using fat stores for energy. That's how weight loss happens on the Keto.

BEAUTY TIPS FROM KETO PRODUCTS

We all know that beauty comes from inside. And we talk so much about what is good to eat to be healthy and beautiful, that we completely forget that those good foods that we take inside can also be used on the outside. I mean natural, homemade, cosmetics of course. In this section we are going to explore homemade face masks from those top 12 Keto foods! The first ingredient in our top 12 list is egg.

The high use of eggs is approved for any skin type, bearing in mind that with oily skin the whites are used and with dry skin the yolks. Egg masks have anti-aging effect and help smooth out the wrinkles.

The egg yolks contain:

- Choline – produces moisturizing and rejuvenating effect
- Iron – nourishes epidermis cells with oxygen
- Vitamin D – slows down aging process
- Vitamin B5 – helps in fighting mimic wrinkles
- Vitamin B12 – allows cell renewal
- Vitamin E – carries antioxidants

The egg whites contain:
- Amino acids – provide face-lifting effect;
- Astringent properties help shrink pores

CHAPTER 2. EGG MASKS

SOFTENING MASK

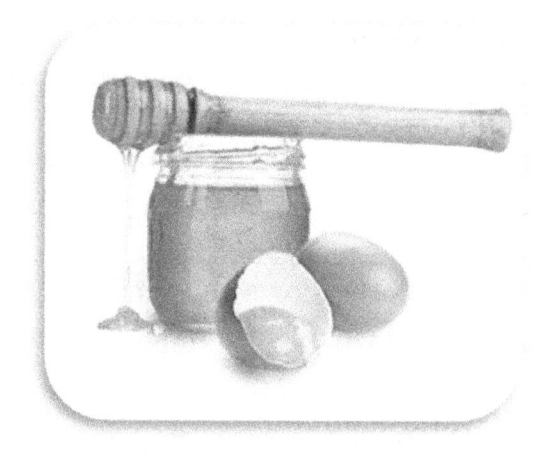

INGREDIENTS

- 1 egg yolk
- 1 Tbsp honey, melted

DIRECTIONS

Mix egg yolk with honey until smooth and apply on face for 20 minutes. Rinse with warm water.

NOURISHING MASK

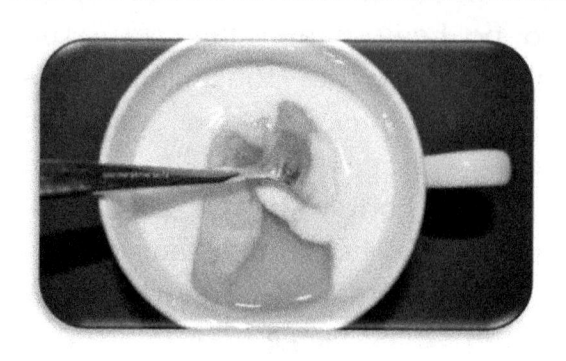

INGREDIENTS

- 1 egg yolk
- 1 Tbsp honey, melted
- 1 tsp yogurt
- 1 tsp butter

DIRECTIONS

Mix egg yolk with butter, yogurt and honey until smooth and apply on face for 20 minutes. Rinse with warm water.

ANTIAGING MASK

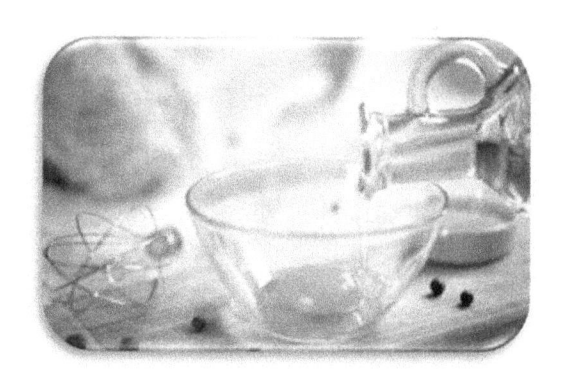

INGREDIENTS

- 1 egg yolk
- 1 Tbsp olive oil

DIRECTIONS

Mix egg yolk with olive oil until smooth and apply on face for 20 minutes. Rinse with warm water.

TONIC MASK

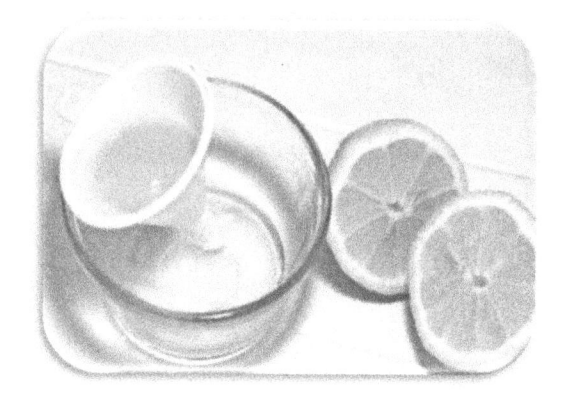

INGREDIENTS

- 1 egg white
- 1 Tbsp lemon juice

DIRECTIONS

Beat egg white until foamy, add 1 Tbsp lemon juice and apply on face for 10 minutes. Rinse with cold water.

CLEANSING MASK

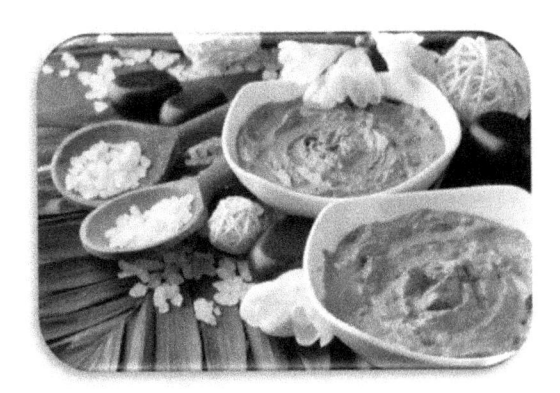

INGREDIENTS

- *1 egg white*
- *1 Tbsp cosmetic clay*
- *Warm water*

DIRECTIONS

1. Add enough warm water to clay to make a spreadable paste.
2. Beat egg white until foamy, add clay and apply on face for 20 minutes. Rinse with cold water.
3. Apply face cream.

ANTIAGING MASK FOR DRY SKIN

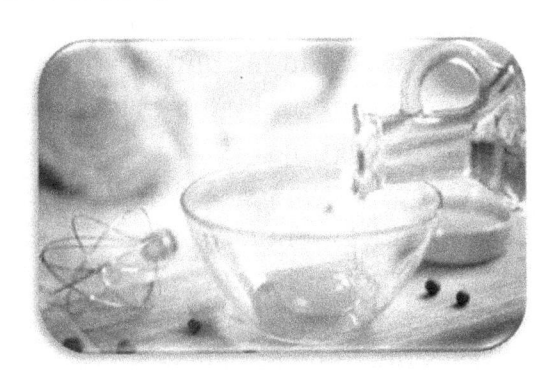

INGREDIENTS

- *1 egg white*
- *2-3 drops lemon juice*
- *1 tsp oatmeal*

DIRECTIONS

1. Beat egg white until foamy; add lemon juice and oatmeal to make a spreadable paste. Apply on face for 15 minutes.
2. Rinse with warm water.

CHAPTER 3. AVOCADO MASKS

Another popular keto ingredient is avocado. The secret of avocado is that the number of microelements, minerals, fats, vitamins and other micronutrients outweigh any other product. Avocado flesh is a great natural antioxidant and moisturizer. Cosmetic benefits for the skin have moisturizing, softening, wound- healing, composing and regenerating effects. The avocado contains:

- Potassium, Calcium, Sodium, Phosphorus, Copper, Iron, Magnesium and others;
- Vitamin E in abundance;
- Vitamins A, B2, B3, B6, C, D, E, F, K, P

AVOCADO MASK FOR DRY SKIN

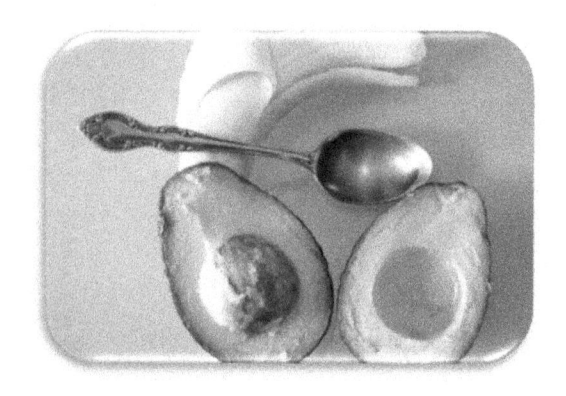

INGREDIENTS

- *1 Tbsp avocado flesh*
- *1 Tbsp banana*
- *1 egg yolk*
- *1 tsp honey*

DIRECTIONS

1. Mix egg yolk with avocado, banana and honey until smooth and apply on face for 20 minutes.
2. Rinse with warm water.

AVOCADO MASK FOR OILY SKIN

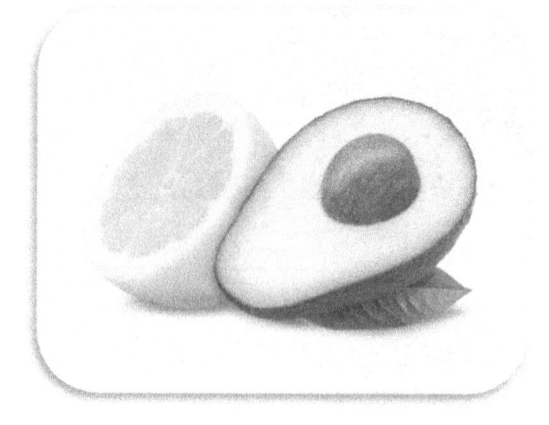

INGREDIENTS

- *1 Tbsp avocado flesh*
- *1 egg yolk*
- *1 tsp lemon juice*

DIRECTIONS

1. Mix egg yolk with avocado and lemon juice until smooth and apply on face for 20 minutes.
2. Rinse with warm water.

AVOCADO MASK FOR FLAKY SKIN

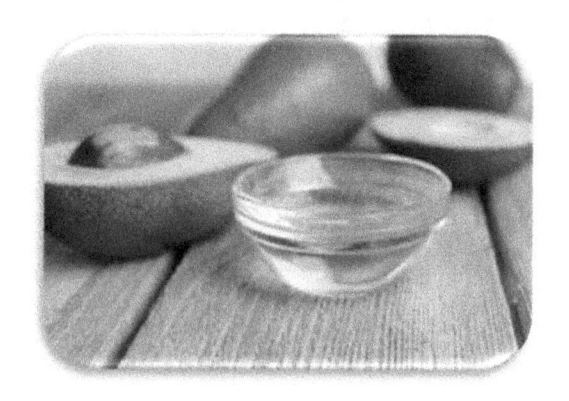

INGREDIENTS

- *3 tsp avocado flesh*
- *1 tsp olive oil*

DIRECTIONS

1. Mix avocado and olive oil until smooth and apply on face for 20 minutes.
2. Rinse with warm water.

CHAPTER 4. RECIPES
EGG RECIPES

OMELET IN A CUP

SERVINGS: 1 | PREP TIME: 3 min. | COOK TIME: 25 min.

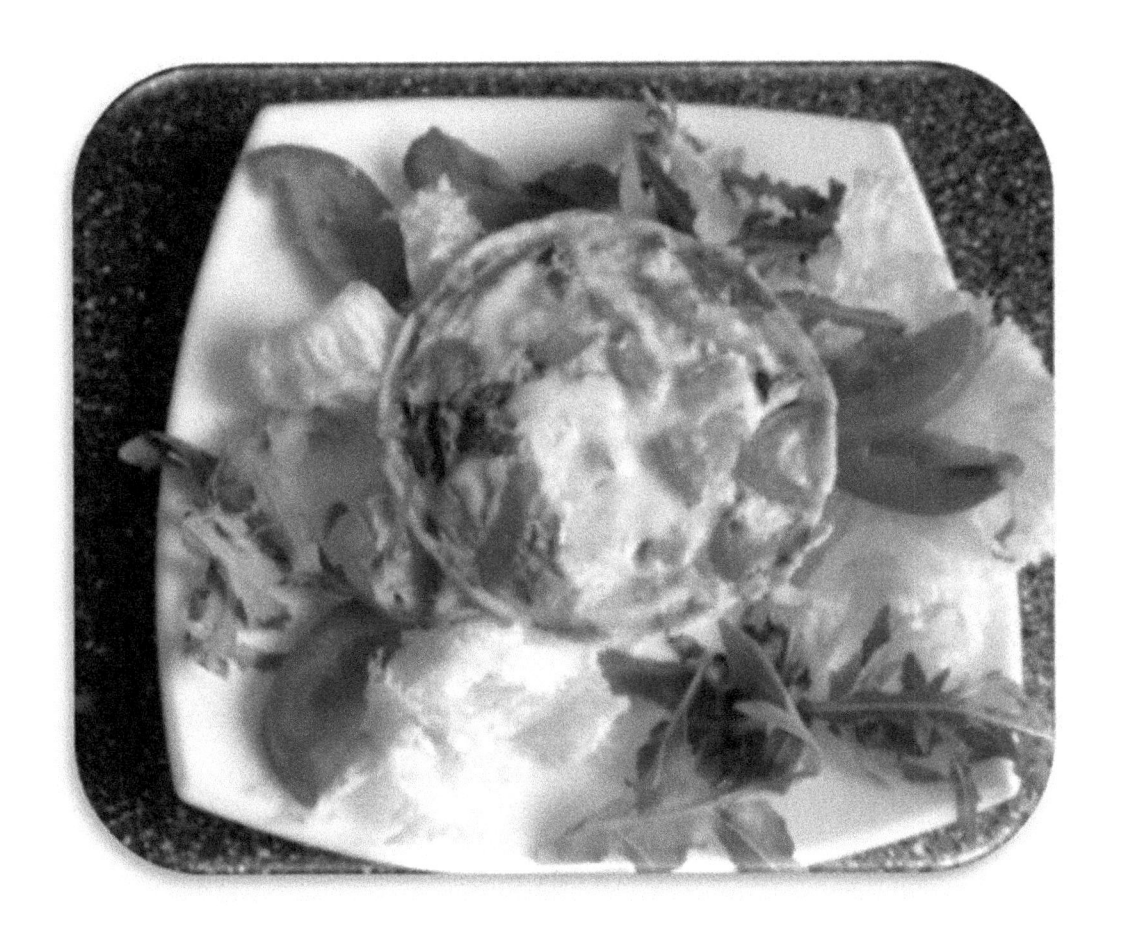

CARBS: 6.7 g | FAT: 18.3 g | PROTEIN: 20 g | CALORIES: 276

INGREDIENTS

- *2 eggs*
- *1.3 oz hard cheese, cubed*
- *1 tomato, chopped*
- *½ tsp Dijon mustard*
- *½ tsp dried parsley*
- *Pinch of garlic powder*
- *Salt to taste*

DIRECTIONS

1. Beat eggs and add cheese, ½ tomato. Season with spices.
2. Pour the egg mix into oven proof cup (bowl/muffin tin) and bake at 356F for 20-30 min.
3. Serve with the remaining fresh tomato and Dijon mustard.

GOAT CHEESE FRITTATA

SERVINGS: 8 | PREP TIME: 3 min. | COOK TIME: 25 min.

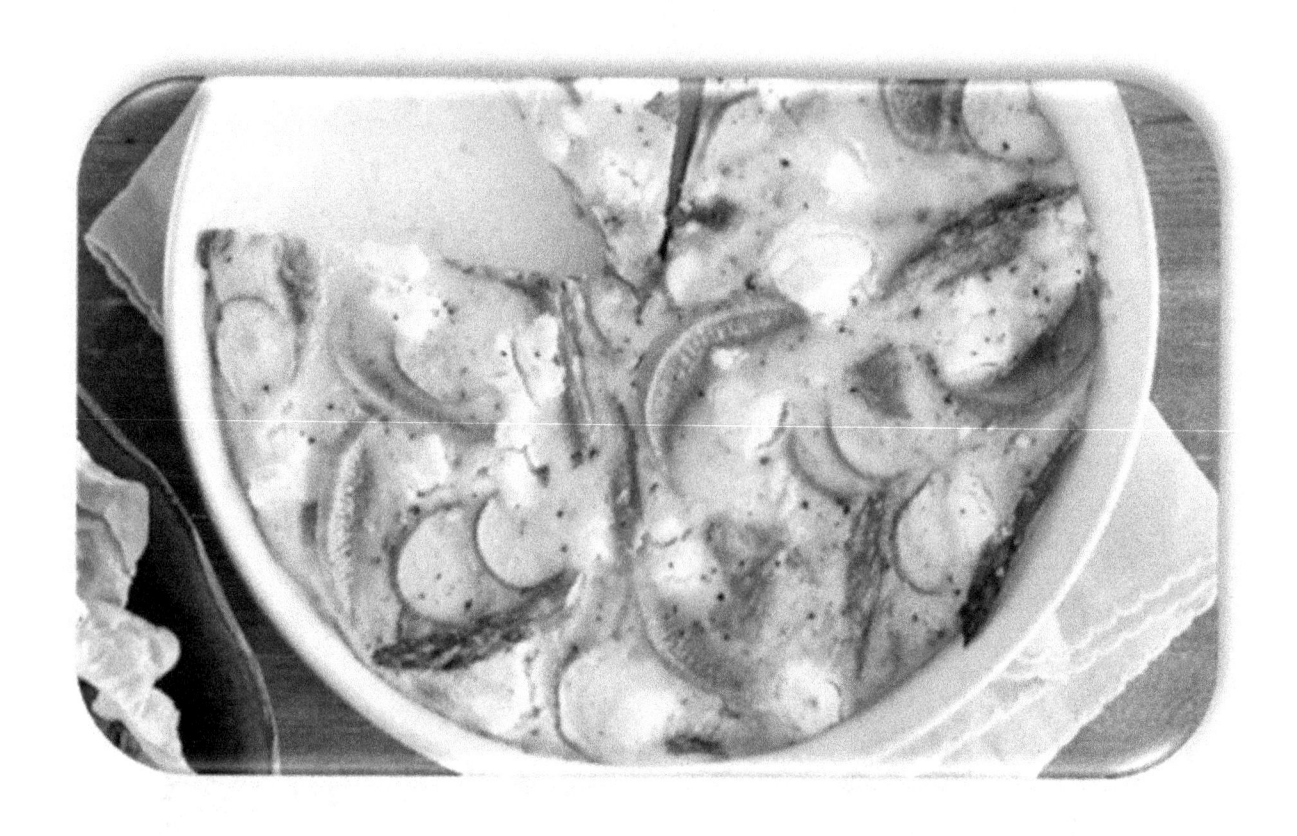

CARBS: 3 g | FAT: 16.2 g | PROTEIN: 12.2 g | CALORIES: 216

INGREDIENTS

- 8 eggs
- 3 oz ham, chopped
- 4 oz goat cheese
- ½ lb asparagus, trimmed, sliced
- 4 scallions, sliced
- 1 garlic clove
- ¾ cup heavy cream
- 2 Tbsp butter
- Salt and pepper to taste

DIRECTIONS

1. Beat eggs and add ham and cream. Season with salt and pepper.
2. Melt butter in a skillet and sauté asparagus up to 4 minutes until crisp tender.
3. Add scallions and garlic and sauté up to 2 minutes until fragrant.
4. Pour egg mixture over vegetables and cook up to 4 minutes until eggs are well cooked. Sprinkle with goat cheese.
5. Bake in the oven for 15 minutes at 350°F.

SQUASH FRITTATA

SERVINGS: 4 | PREP TIME: 10 min. | COOK TIME: 30 min.

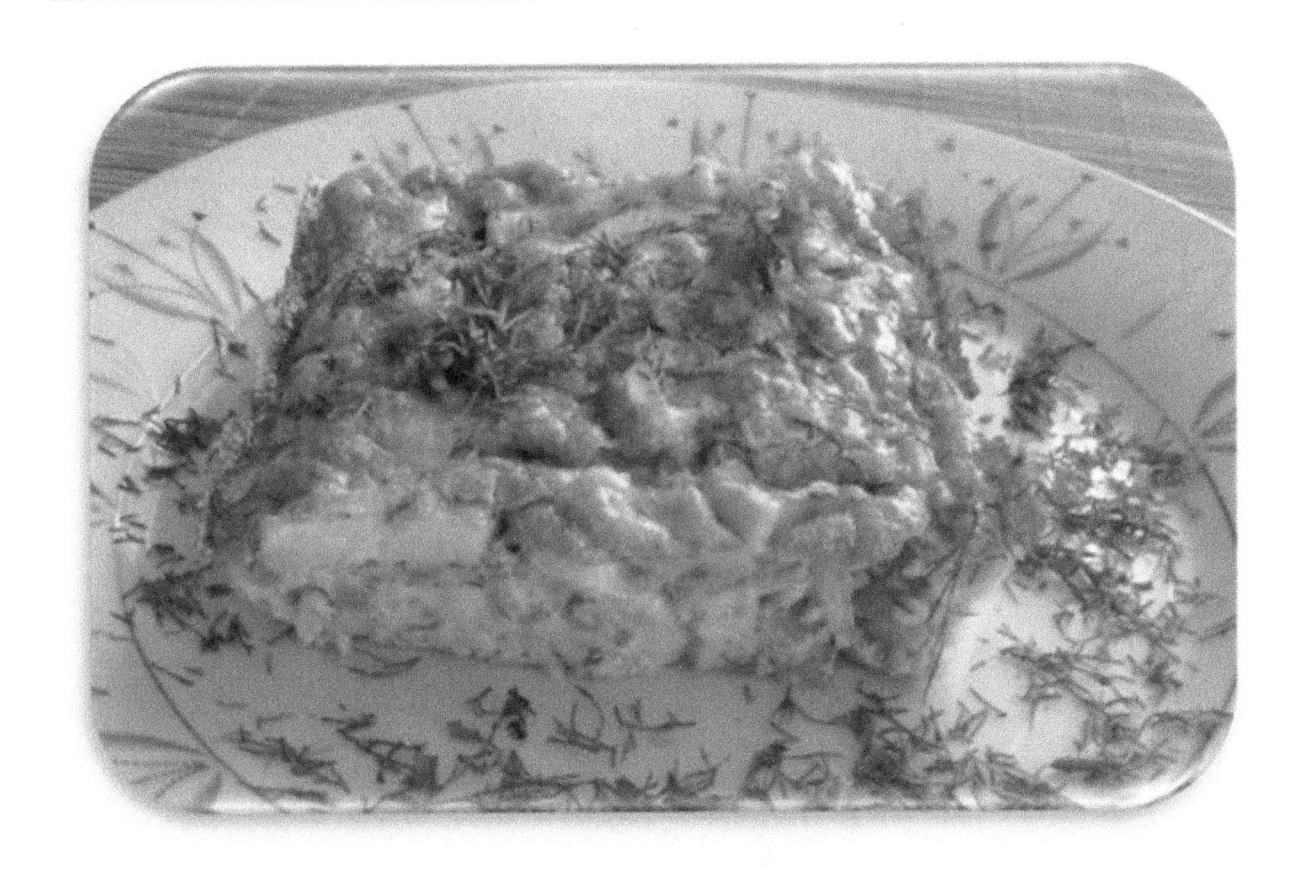

CARBS: 7 g | FAT: 3.7 g | PROTEIN: 5.2 g | CALORIES: 49

INGREDIENTS

- *5 eggs, beaten*
- *1 onion, minced*
- *8 oz summer squash, peeled, cubed*
- *Fresh dill, minced*
- *Olive oil for frying*
- *Salt & pepper to taste*

DIRECTIONS

1. Fry the onions for 2-3 minutes in the olive oil.
2. Add the cubed squash and let cook for 5 minutes. Season with salt.
3. Using a blender beat eggs with salt and dill.
4. Add squash to a greased baking pan, pour in the egg mixture.
5. Bake at 356°F for about 30 minutes until eggs are not runny.

SCOTCH QUAIL EGGS

SERVINGS: 12 | PREP TIME: 10 min. | COOK TIME: 15 min.

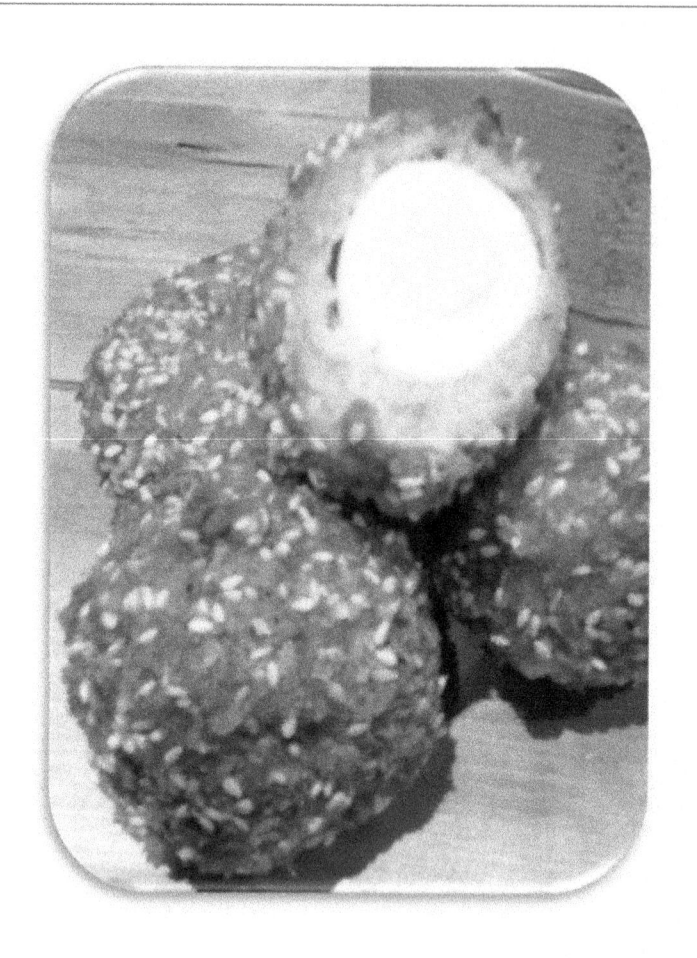

CARBS: 4 g | FAT: 5.9 g | PROTEIN: 6.4 g | CALORIES: 97

INGREDIENTS

- *12 quail eggs*
- *2 thick sausages, meat squeezed out, skin discarded,*
- *2 sprigs thyme*
- *1 chicken egg, beaten*
- *Sesame seeds*
- *Olive oil for frying*

DIRECTIONS

1. Boil the quail eggs for 2 minutes, cool down and peel.
2. In one bowl beat a raw chicken egg. Place the sesame seeds into another bowl.
3. Divide the sausage mixture into 12 portions, Shape it around the quail eggs, and carefully roll it into balls.
4. Dip into the beaten chicken egg and then coat with sesame seeds.
5. Fry in a deep pan with olive oil for 1-2 minutes until golden.
6. Then bake in the oven at 356°F for 5 minutes.

MEDITERRANEAN DELIVED EGGS

SERVINGS: 12 | PREP TIME: 5 min. | COOK TIME: 15 min.

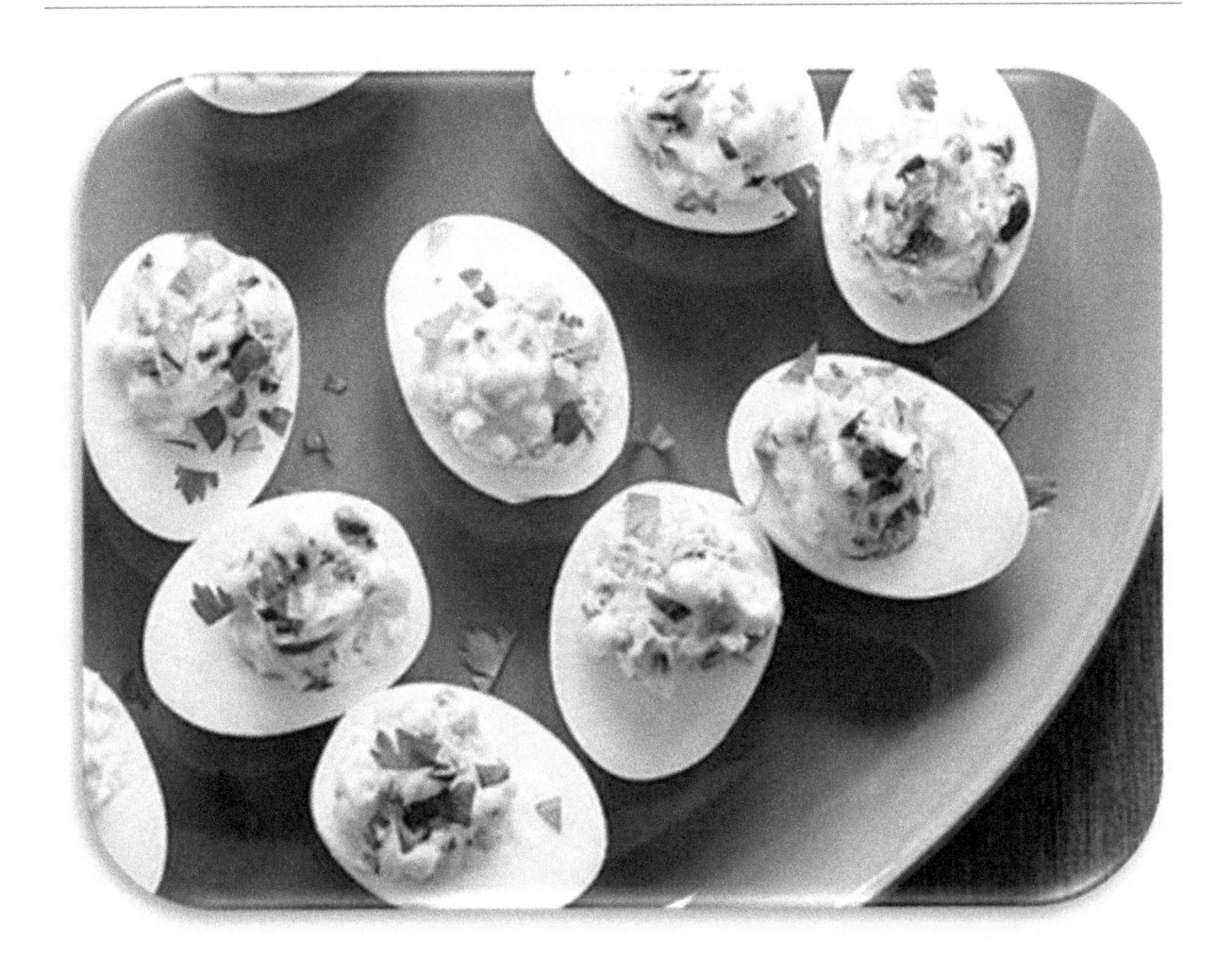

CARBS: 3.5 g | FAT: 5.4 g | PROTEIN: 10 g | CALORIES: 103

INGREDIENTS

- 12 eggs, hard-boiled, peeled
- 5 anchovy fillets, chopped
- 6 Tbsp sun-dried tomatoes, chopped finely
- 6 Tbsp Greek yogurt
- 2 Tbsp chives, chopped
- 4 tsp lemon juice
- 12 oregano leaves
- Pepper to taste

DIRECTIONS

1. Halve each egg and remove the yolks.
2. Mash the yolks. Combine with tomatoes, chives, anchovies, yogurt and lemon juice.
3. Fill each egg half and sprinkle with oregano leaves.

EGG PASTE

SERVINGS: 4 | PREP TIME: 15 min. | COOK TIME: 1 h. 15 min.

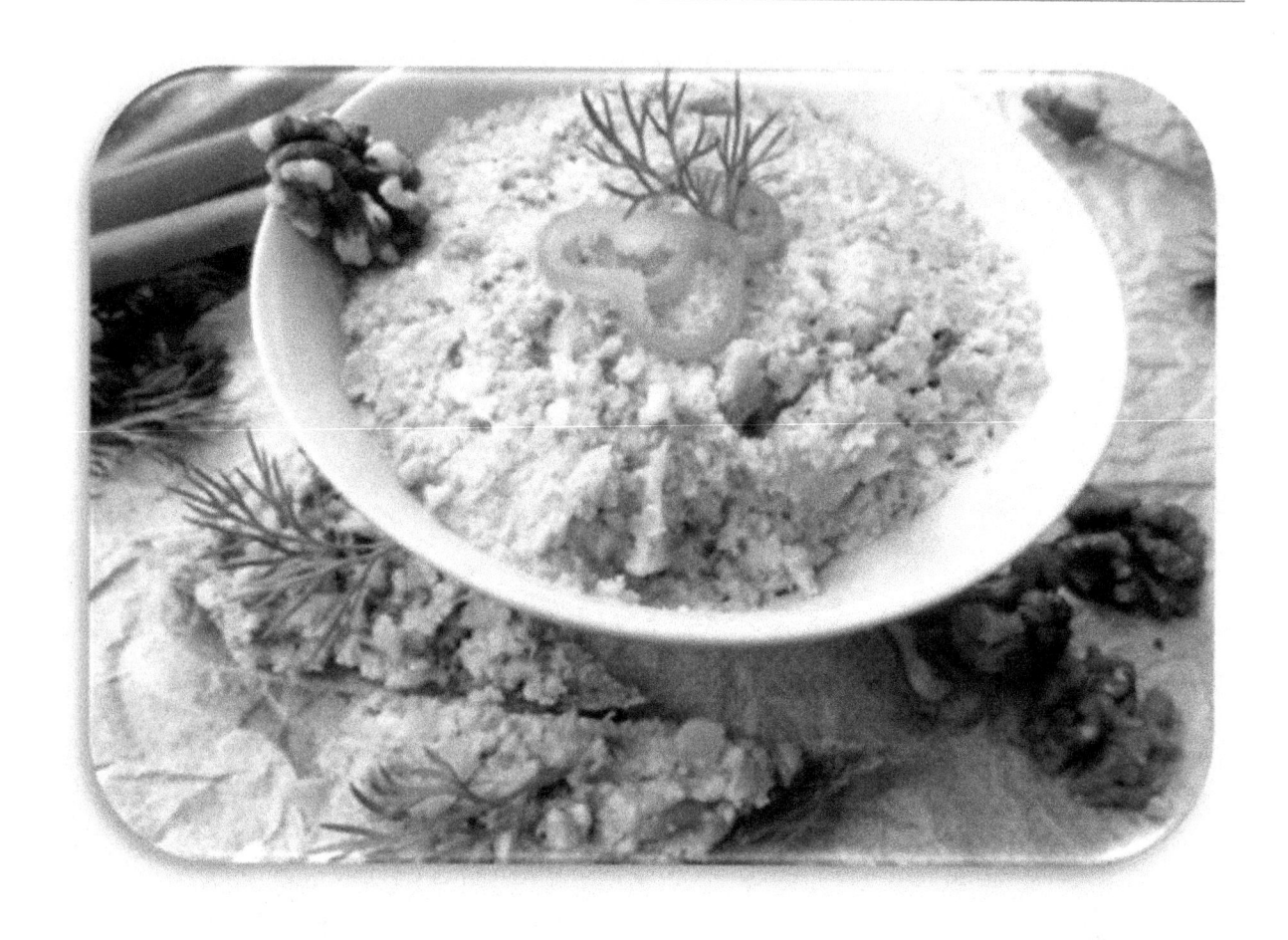

CARBS: 3.5 g | FAT: 17.3 g | PROTEIN: 4.7 g | CALORIES: 187

INGREDIENTS

- *2 eggs, hard-boiled, peeled, chopped*
- *1 Tbsp butter*
- *1 oz walnuts*
- *1 garlic clove*
- *1 onion, chopped finely*
- *2 Tbsp olive oil*
- *Salt and pepper to taste*

DIRECTIONS

1. Combine the butter and olive oil
2. Fry the onions in butter and olive oil until golden.
3. In a blender mince together eggs, walnuts, onions and garlic.
4. Season with salt and pepper. Transfer to a bowl and refrigerate for 1–2 hours.

MUSHROOMS STUFFED WITH EGGS

SERVINGS: 4 | PREP TIME: 15 min. | COOK TIME: 15 min.

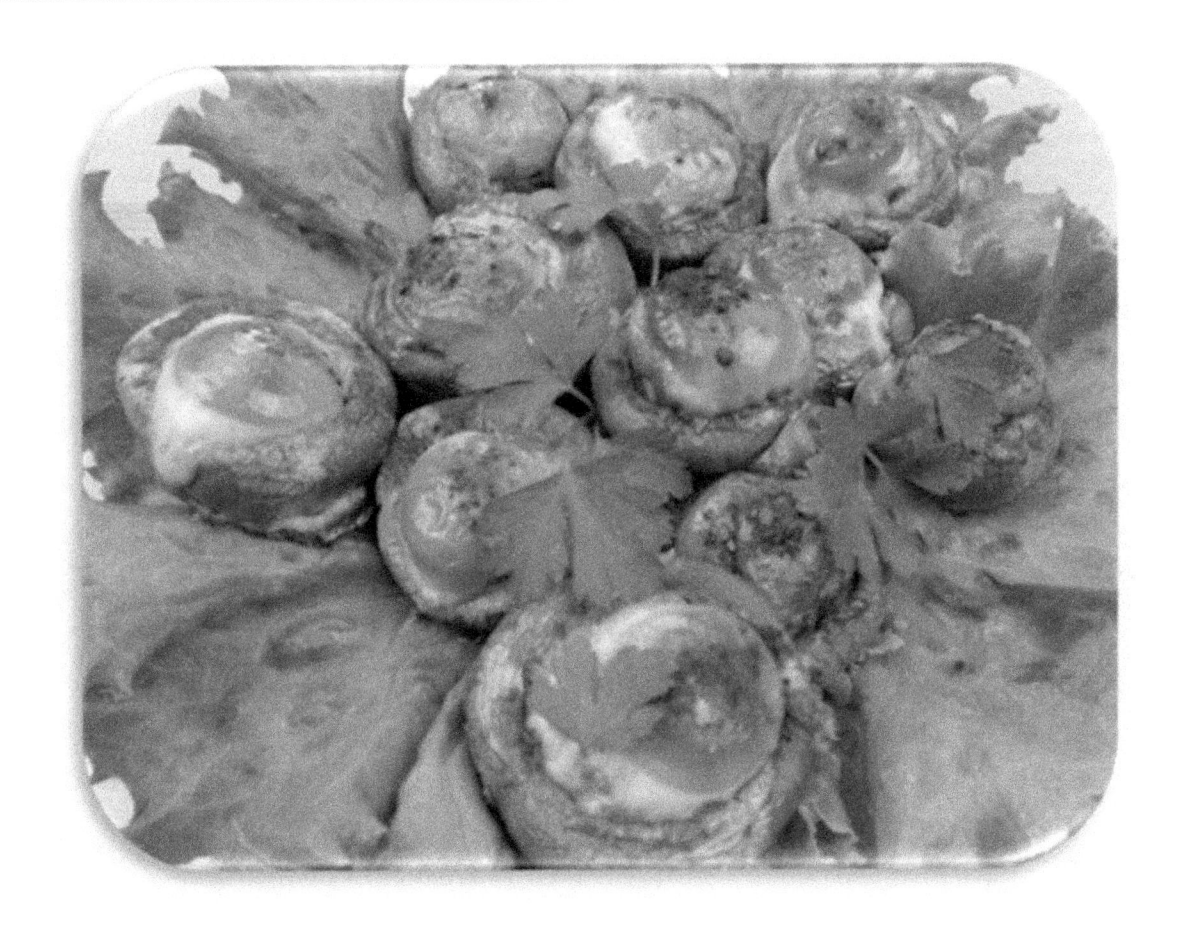

CARBS: 14 g | FAT: 8.8 g | PROTEIN: 18.2 g | CALORIES: 192

INGREDIENTS

- *15 quail eggs, raw*
- *15 white mushrooms, rinsed, stems removed and reserved*
- *1 onion, chopped*
- *¼ cup hard cheese, grated*
- *Olive oil for frying*
- *Salt and pepper to taste*

DIRECTIONS

1. Chop the mushroom stems. Add to a pan preheated with olive oil and fry together with the chopped onions.
2. Season with salt and pepper.
3. Fill the caps and sprinkle with cheese. Crack an egg into each mushroom cap. Season with salt.
4. Bake for 15 minutes at 356F.

BROCCOLI OMELET

SERVINGS: 4 | PREP TIME: 5 min. | COOK TIME: 15 min.

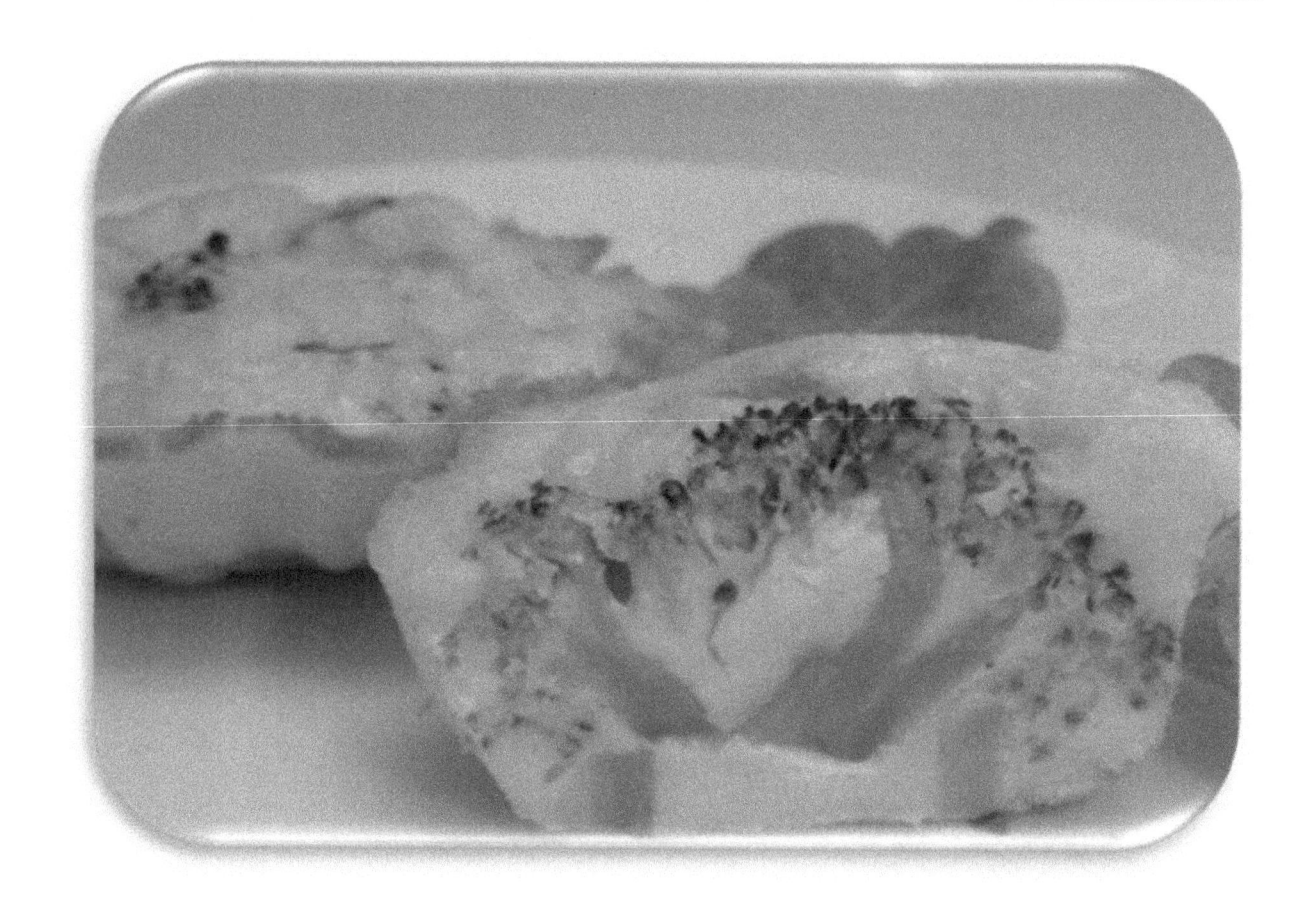

CARBS: 1 g | FAT: 2.8 g | PROTEIN: 2.4 g | CALORIES: 39

INGREDIENTS

- *2 eggs*
- *4 broccoli florets*
- *2 Tbsp sour cream*
- *1-2 tsp keto flour (almond or coconut)*
- *Salt and pepper to taste*
- *Butter for greasing*

DIRECTIONS

1. Beat the eggs with the sour cream and salt.
2. Add flour and blend well.
3. Prepare 4 muffin molds by greasing them with some butter.
4. Add one broccoli floret into each cup and fill with the omelet mixture.
5. Bake for 15-20 minutes at 374°F.

EGGS FLORENTINE

SERVINGS: 4 | PREP TIME: 5 min. | COOK TIME: 30 min.

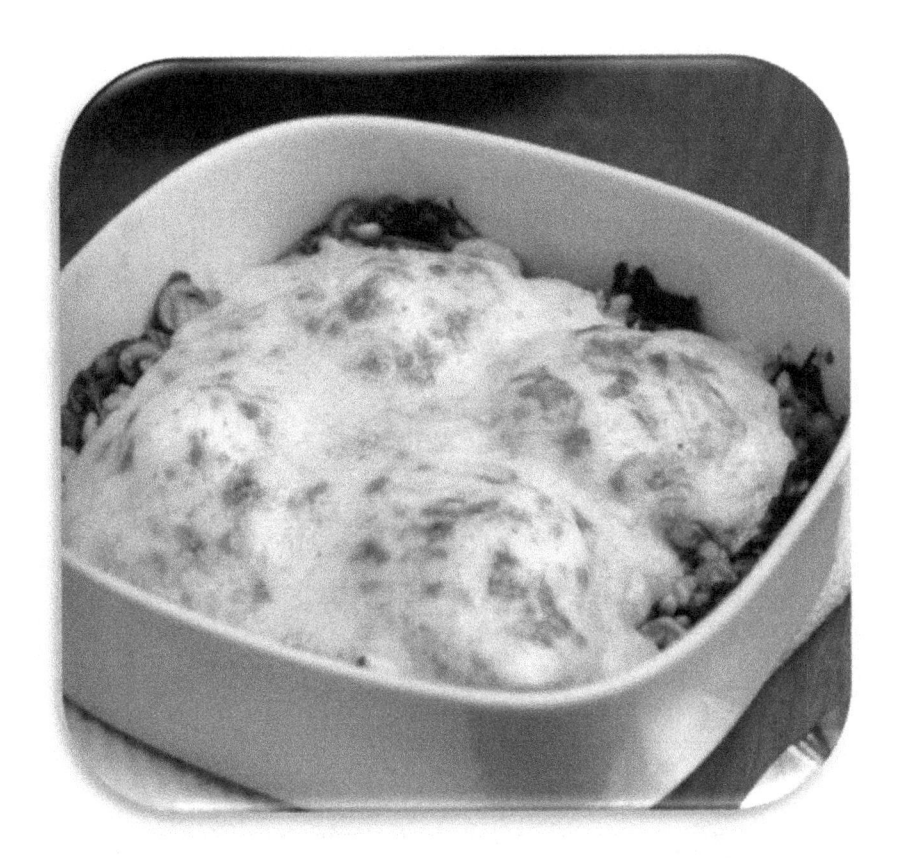

CARBS: 14 g | FAT: 8.4 g | PROTEIN: 13 g | CALORIES: 183

INGREDIENTS

- 4 eggs
- 2 cups spinach leaves, boiled until soft (2-3 min.)
- 3 spring onions, chopped
- 10–12 white mushrooms, sliced
- 4 Tbsp butter
- 1 cup sour cream
- 1 cup Cheddar, grated
- 1 tsp mustard
- Salt and pepper to taste
- Butter for greasing

DIRECTIONS

1. Prepare a baking dish by greasing with some butter. Arrange spinach leaves at the bottom of it.
2. Heat 1 Tbsp butter in a frying pan and add the mushrooms. Cook, stirring, for 2 minutes. Add the spring onions and cook for 2 more minutes. Season with salt and pepper.
3. Spread the mushrooms and spring onions over the spinach layer.
4. Fill a saucepan with ½ inch water and bring to a simmer. Lightly coat four poaching cups with nonstick cooking spray and crack an egg into each cup. Place the cups in the simmering water, cover and cook until the whites are firm and the yolks are glazed over but still soft, about 3 minutes.
5. Carefully transfer the eggs to the baking dish on top of the mushrooms.
6. Combine sour cream with mustard and mix well. Pour over the eggs and sprinkle with the cheese.
7. Bake for 20–25 minutes at 374°F.

EGG AND SHRIMP SALAD

SERVINGS: 4 | PREP TIME: 5 min. | COOK TIME: 30 min.

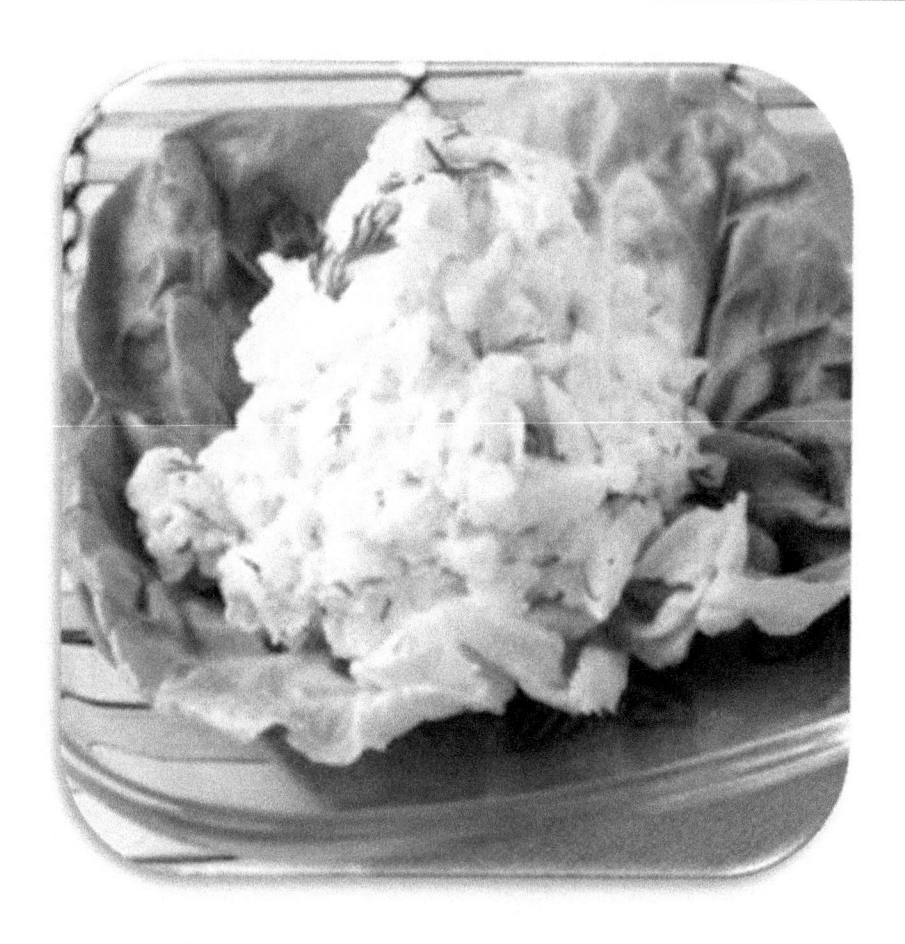

CARBS: 1.6 g | FAT: 17.5 g | PROTEIN: 30.3 g | CALORIES: 292

INGREDIENTS

- 4 eggs, hard-boiled, peeled, chopped
- 1 lb shrimp, cooked, peeled, deveined, chopped
- 4 lettuce leaves
- 1 sprig dill, chopped
- 4 Tbsp mayonnaise
- 1 tsp Dijon mustard
- Salt and pepper to taste

DIRECTIONS

1. Combine all ingredients in a salad bowl and toss well with the mayonnaise and mustard.
2. Serve on lettuce leaves.

BACON RECIPES

BACON AND EGG FAT BOMBS

SERVINGS: 6 | PREP TIME: 40 min. | COOK TIME: 15 min.

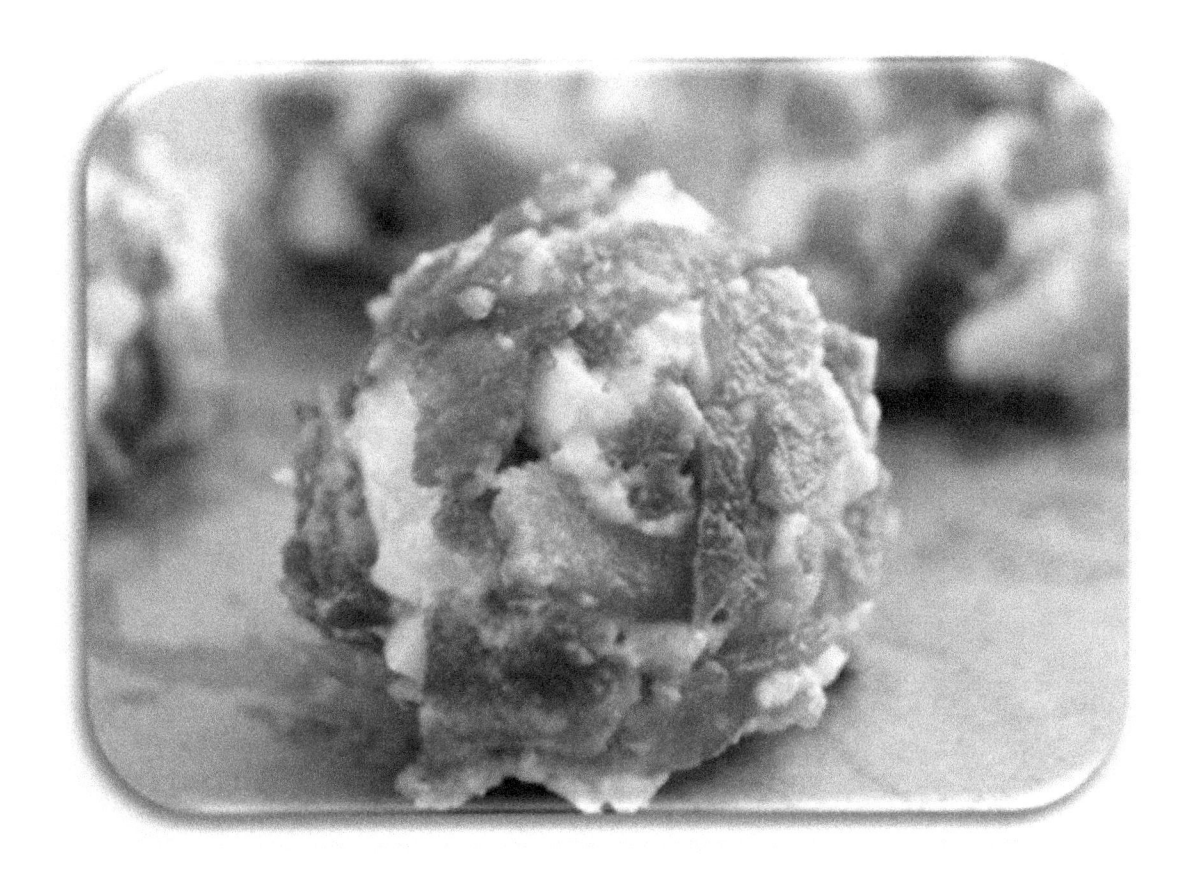

CARBS: 0.2 g | FAT: 18.4 g | PROTEIN: 5 g | CALORIES: 185

INGREDIENTS

- *2 large eggs, hard-boiled, cut into quarters*
- *¼ cup butter*
- *2 Tbsp mayonnaise*
- *4 large slices bacon*
- *Salt, pepper to taste*

DIRECTIONS

1. Preheat the oven to 375 °F.
2. Cook the bacon strips on a baking tray for 15 minutes. Reserve the grease.
3. Cut the butter into pieces and add the quartered eggs. Mash with a fork to mix.
4. Add the remaining ingredients except the bacon and mix. Pour in the bacon grease. Mix well. Refrigerate for 20–30 minutes.
5. Crumble the bacon. Create 6 balls from the egg mixture and roll each ball in the bacon crumbs.
6. Serve.

FRIED BACON AND CABBAGE

SERVINGS: 6 | PREP TIME: 10 min. | COOK TIME: 50 min.

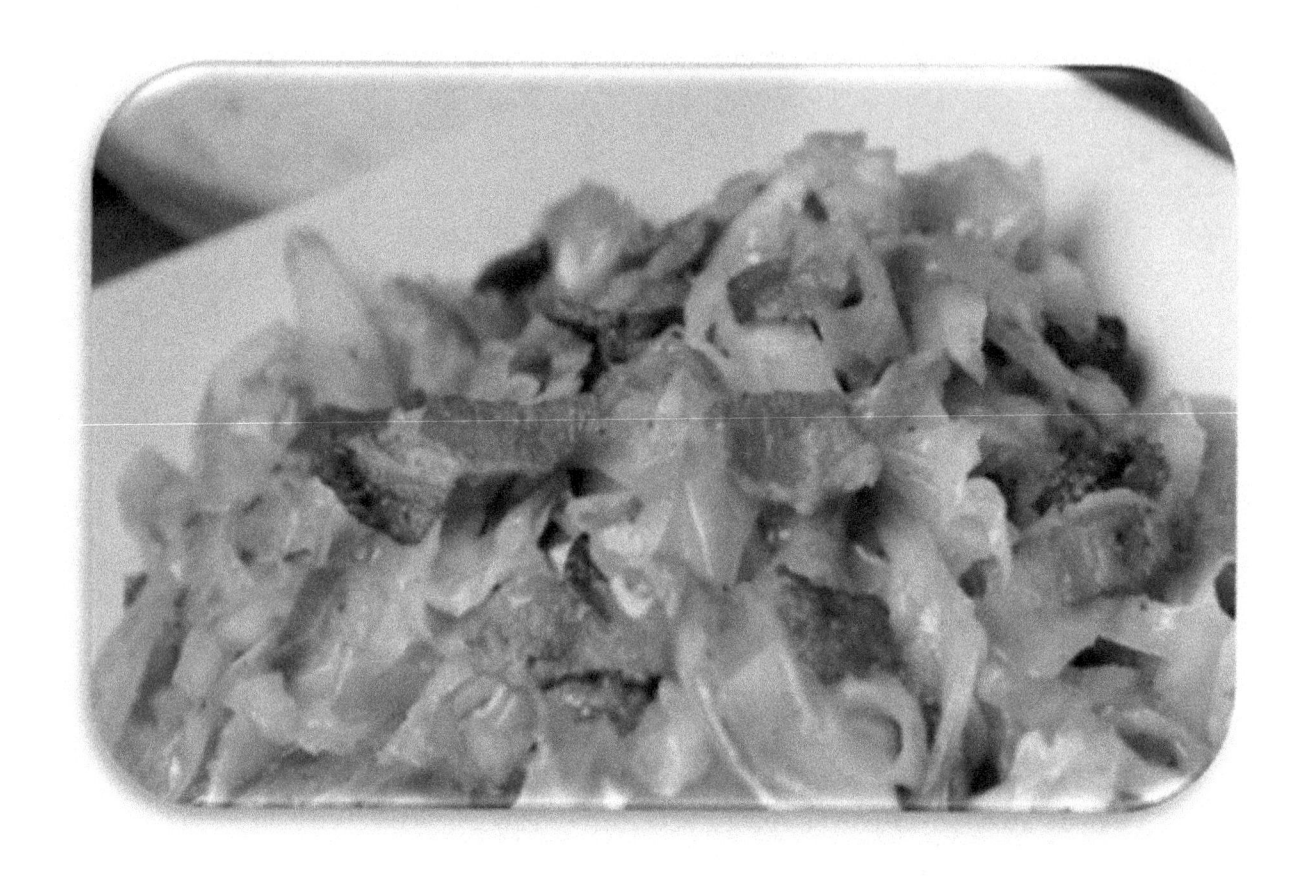

CARBS: 9 g | FAT: 25 g | PROTEIN: 8.5 g | CALORIES: 298

INGREDIENTS

- *6 slices bacon, chopped*
- *1 head cabbage, cored, chopped*
- *1 onion, chopped*
- *3 garlic cloves, minced*
- *Onion & garlic powder to taste*
- *Salt & pepper to taste*

DIRECTIONS

1. Cook the bacon until crisp, remove from pan, reserving 2 Tbsp grease.
2. Using the reserved bacon grease sauté onions until soft, add garlic and sauté for 1 more minute.
3. Stir in the cabbage and cook for 5 minutes. Season with salt, pepper, onion and garlic powder.
4. Reduce heat and let simmer for 30 minutes on low.
5. Mix in the bacon before serving.

BACON WRAPPED CHICKEN

SERVINGS: 4 | PREP TIME: 10 min. | COOK TIME: 30 min.

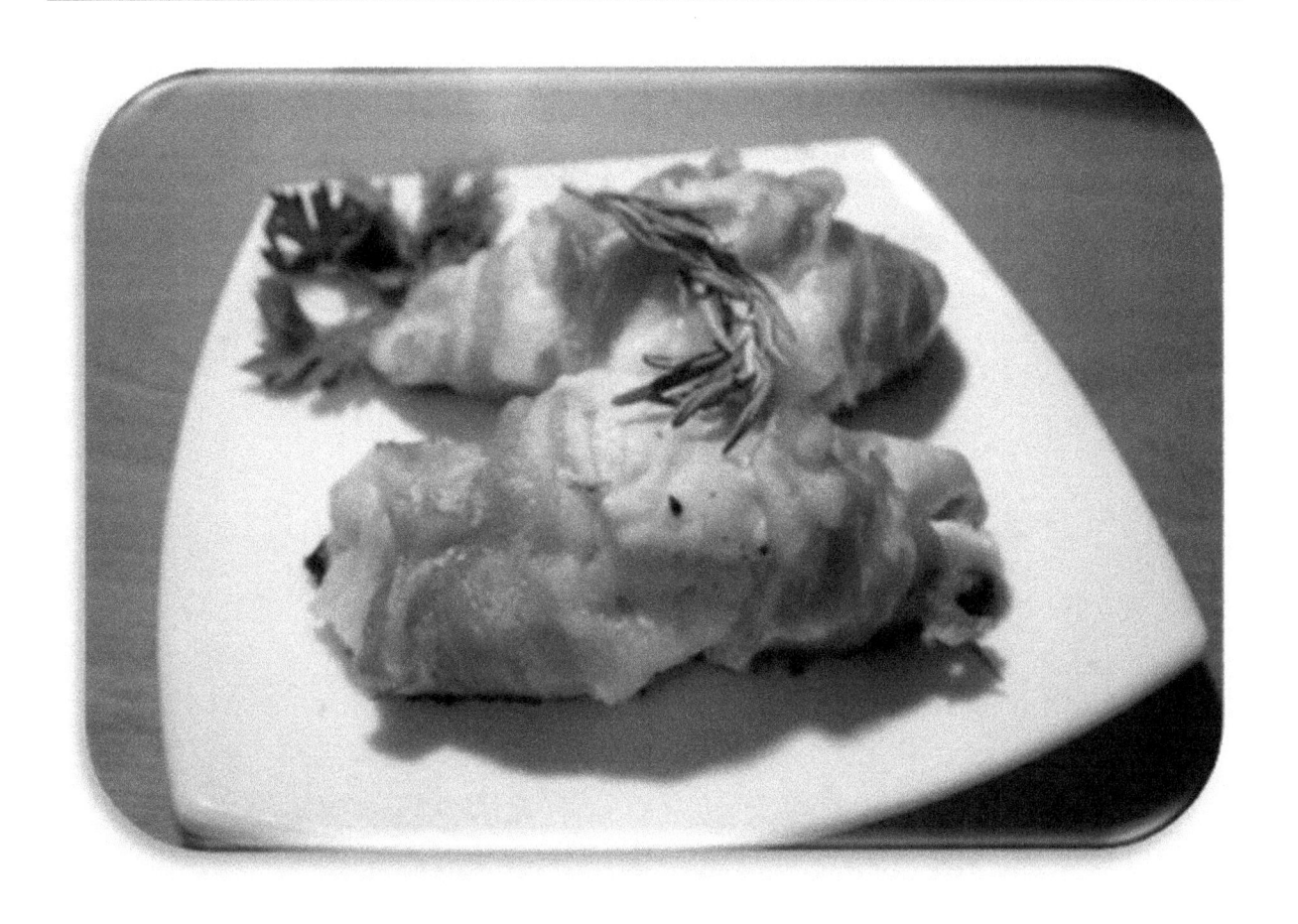

CARBS: 1.5 g | FAT: 7.9 g | PROTEIN: 30.3 g | CALORIES: 206

INGREDIENTS

- 4 slices bacon
- 4 chicken breasts, skinless, rinsed
- 20 oz Mozzarella, cut into strips
- Olive oil for baking
- 1 Tbsp thyme leaves.
- 1 rosemary sprig
- Salt and pepper to taste

DIRECTIONS

1. Make a cut lengthwise (not all the way through) in each chicken breast.
2. Season the chicken with salt and pepper.
3. Insert the Mozzarella strips into the cuts.
4. Wrap chicken breasts with bacon each and secure with toothpicks.
5. Sprinkle with thyme and rosemary to taste.
6. Place onto a baking sheet greased with some olive oil and bake at 392°F for 30 minutes.

BACON WRAPPED MOZZARELLA

SERVINGS: 4 | PREP TIME: 10 min. | COOK TIME: 10 min.

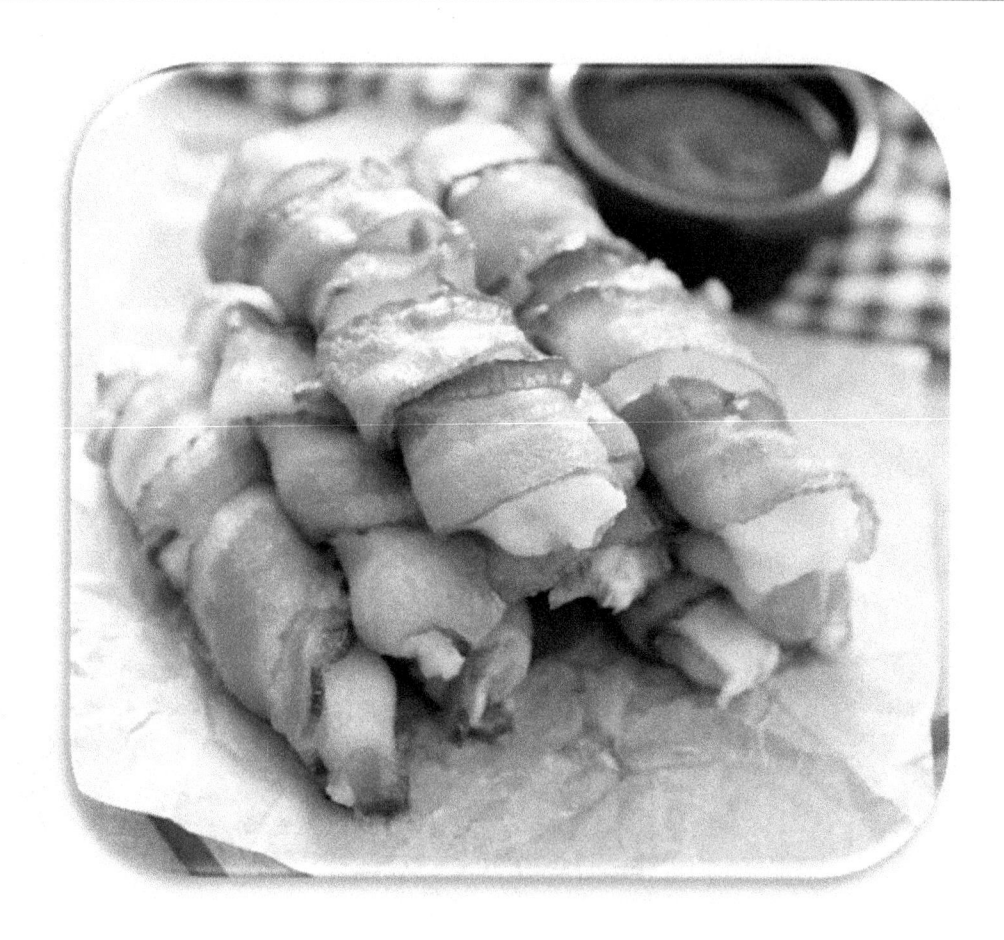

CARBS: 5.4 g | FAT: 122 g | PROTEIN: 39 g | CALORIES: 1301

INGREDIENTS

- *36 slices precooked bacon*
- *12 Mozzarella cheese sticks*
- *Salt and pepper to taste*

DIRECTIONS

1. Wrap a bacon strip around a cheese stick. Wrap another bacon strip until the cheese is completely covered.
2. Place the wrapped Mozzarella on a baking sheet lined with parchment paper.
3. Repeat with the remaining cheese sticks.
4. Bake at 425°F for up to 10 minutes.

BACON TIES

SERVINGS: 4 | PREP TIME: 10 min. | COOK TIME: 25 min.

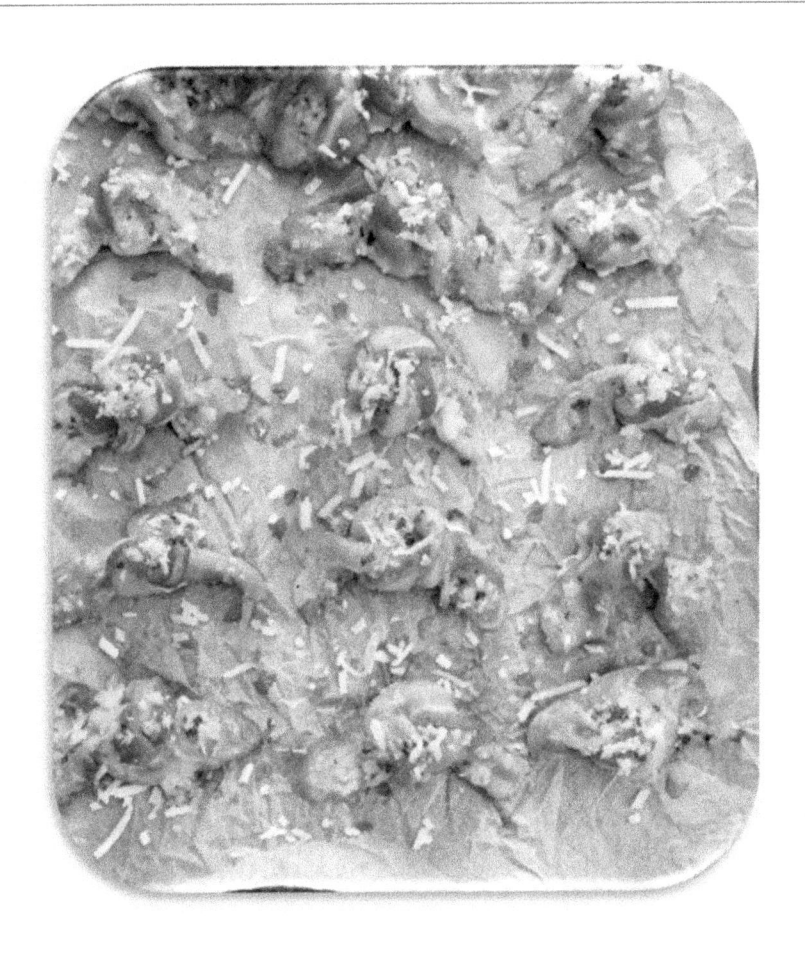

CARBS: 1.3 g | FAT: 33 g | PROTEIN: 30 g | CALORIES: 442

INGREDIENTS

- *16 slices bacon, raw*
- *¼ cup Parmesan, shredded*
- *4 garlic cloves, minced*
- *1 Tbsp parsley, minced*
- *Salt and pepper to taste*

DIRECTIONS

1. Stretch out one slice of bacon and tie into a knot. Then take another slice and tie another knot on top.
2. Repeat with the remaining bacon.
3. Place on a baking sheet lined with parchment paper.
4. Sprinkle with garlic and bake at 400°F up to 15 minutes until crispy.
5. Sprinkle with cheese and parsley and bake for 7 more minutes.

ROMAINE SALAD

SERVINGS: 4 | PREP TIME: 10 min. | COOK TIME: 10 min.

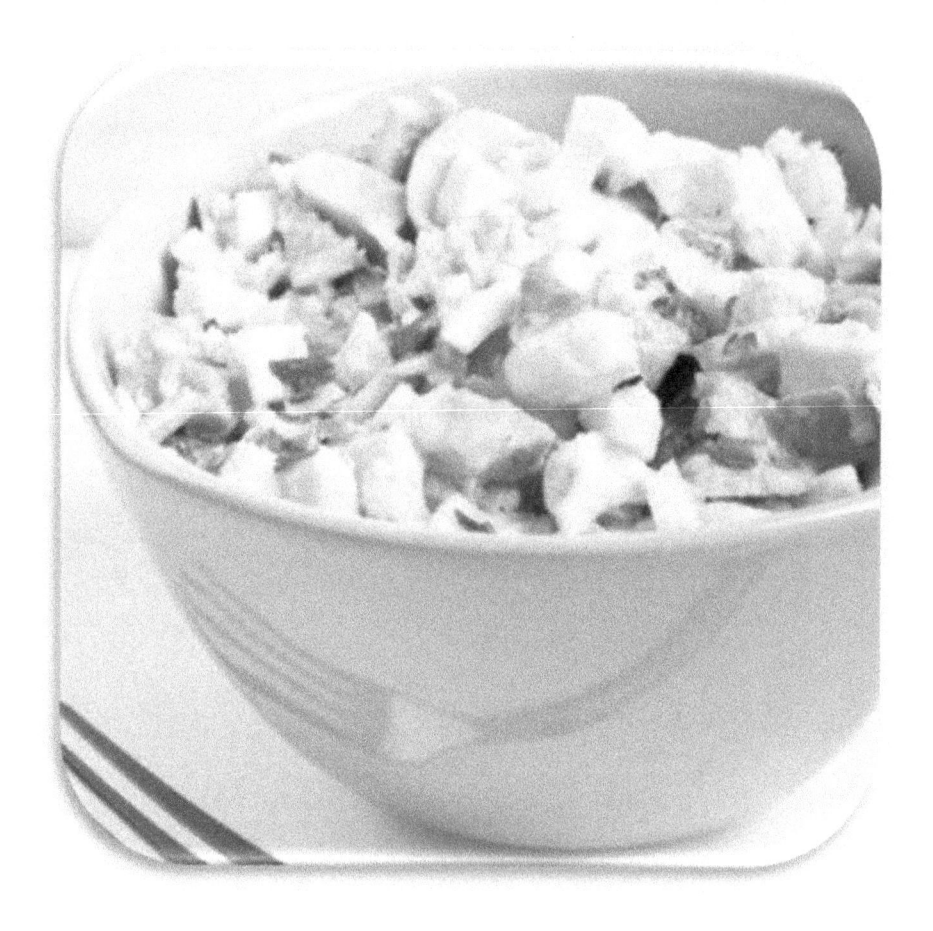

CARBS: 5 g | FAT: 27 g | PROTEIN: 11.7 g | CALORIES: 309

INGREDIENTS

- 4 oz bacon, cut and fried until crisp
- 2 eggs, hard-boiled, chopped
- 1 head Romaine lettuce leaves, chopped
- 2 Tbsp olive oil
- 2 Tbsp red wine vinegar
- ¼ cup shallots, chopped
- Salt to taste
- Olive oil for cooking shallots

DIRECTIONS

1. In the skillet where you fried the bacon add shallots and cook with the remained bacon grease for 2 minutes.
2. Add red wine vinegar to the same skillet with the shallots, season with salt and bring to a boil.
3. In a salad bowl combine chopped eggs, lettuce leaves and bacon. Pour over the warm shallot mixture and mix well.

WARM BACON AND ARUGULA SALAD

SERVINGS: 2 | PREP TIME: 10 min. | COOK TIME: 5 min.

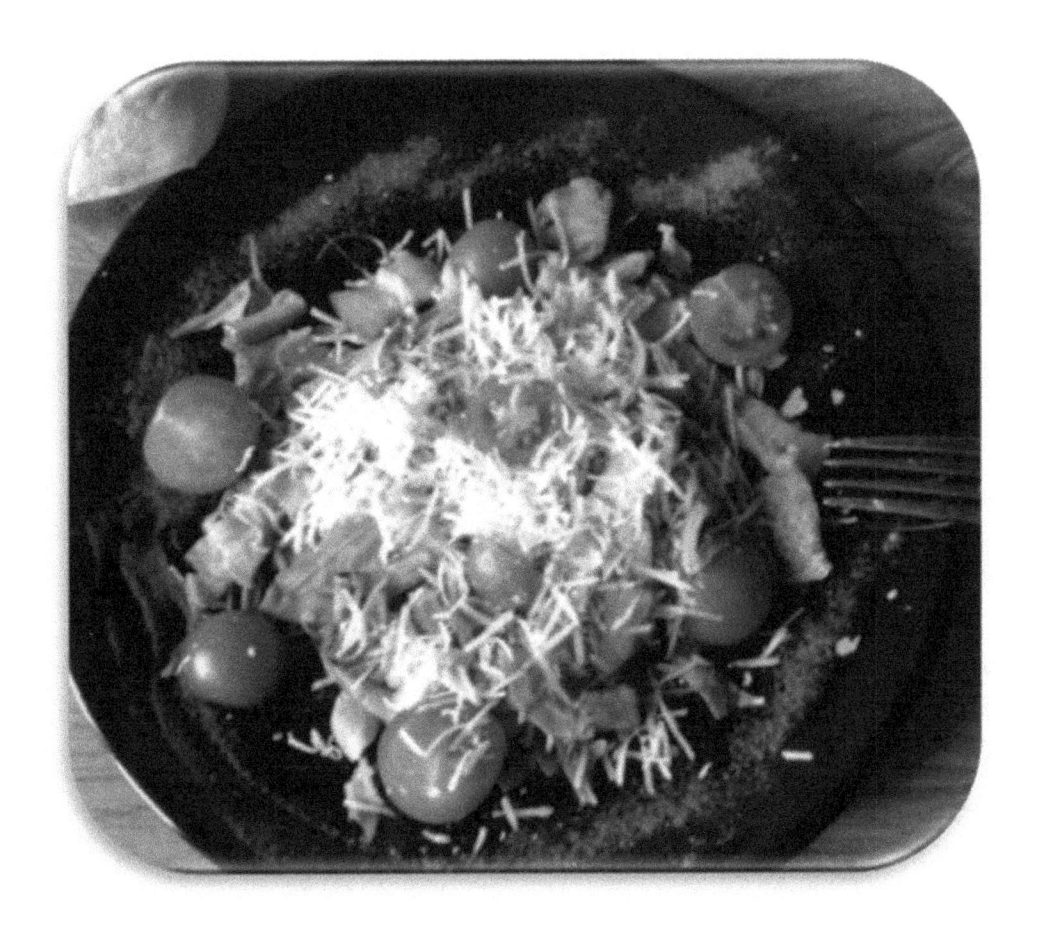

CARBS: 6 g | FAT: 49 g | PROTEIN: 21.7 g | CALORIES: 556

INGREDIENTS

- *4 oz smoked bacon, cut into pieces*
- *8 oz (1 ¼ cups) cherry tomatoes, halved*
- *7 oz arugula, torn*
- *1/3 cup Parmesan, grated*
- *2 Tbsp olive oil*
- *½ Tbsp balsamic vinegar*
- *Salt to taste*

DIRECTIONS

1. Add bacon to a frying pan and cook until golden.
2. Make the salad dressing by mixing ½ tablespoon balsamic vinegar with 2 tablespoons olive oil.
3. Place arugula on serving plates and dress with vinegar & oil mix, add tomatoes, bacon and Parmesan.

BACON SALAD WITH WALNUTS

SERVINGS: 10 | PREP TIME: 10 min. | COOK TIME: 5 min.

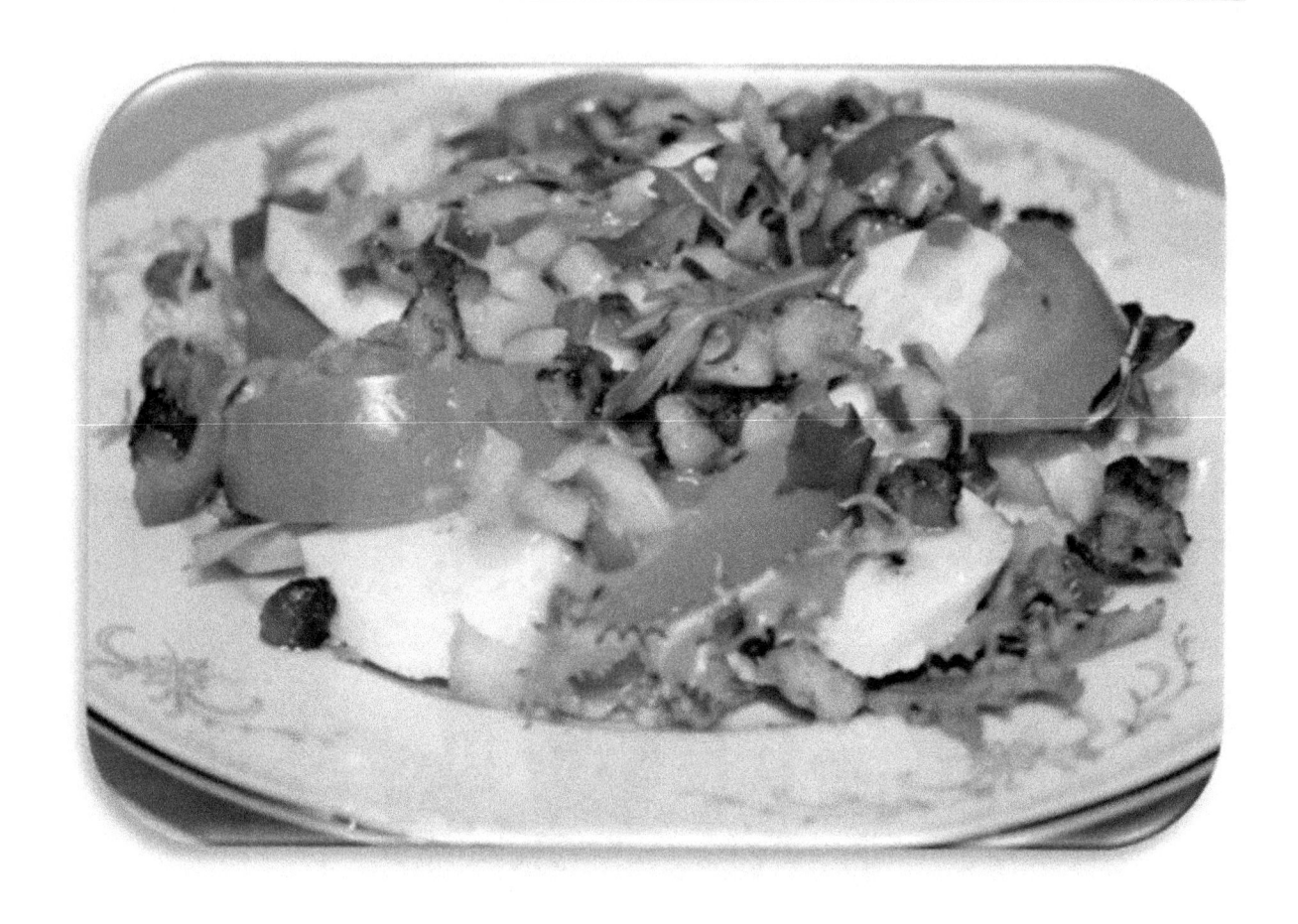

CARBS: 4 g | FAT: 73.4 g | PROTEIN: 24.1 g | CALORIES: 770

INGREDIENTS

- *4 oz bacon, cut into pieces*
- *3.5 oz hard cheese, cubed*
- *2 tomatoes, cubed*
- *15 walnuts, chopped*
- *1 Tbsp capers, sliced*
- *3 garlic cloves*
- *5 Tbsp olive oil*
- *1 Tbsp vinegar*
- *1 Tbsp Dijon mustard*
- *Salt and pepper to taste*

DIRECTIONS

1. Add bacon to a frying pan and cook in olive oil with garlic and black pepper.
2. Remove the bacon and add walnuts.
3. Make the dressing by mixing olive oil with vinegar and mustard.
4. Combine all ingredients and dress. Season with salt and pepper to taste.

BACON AND PEAR SALAD

SERVINGS: 4 | PREP TIME: 10 min. | COOK TIME: 5 min.

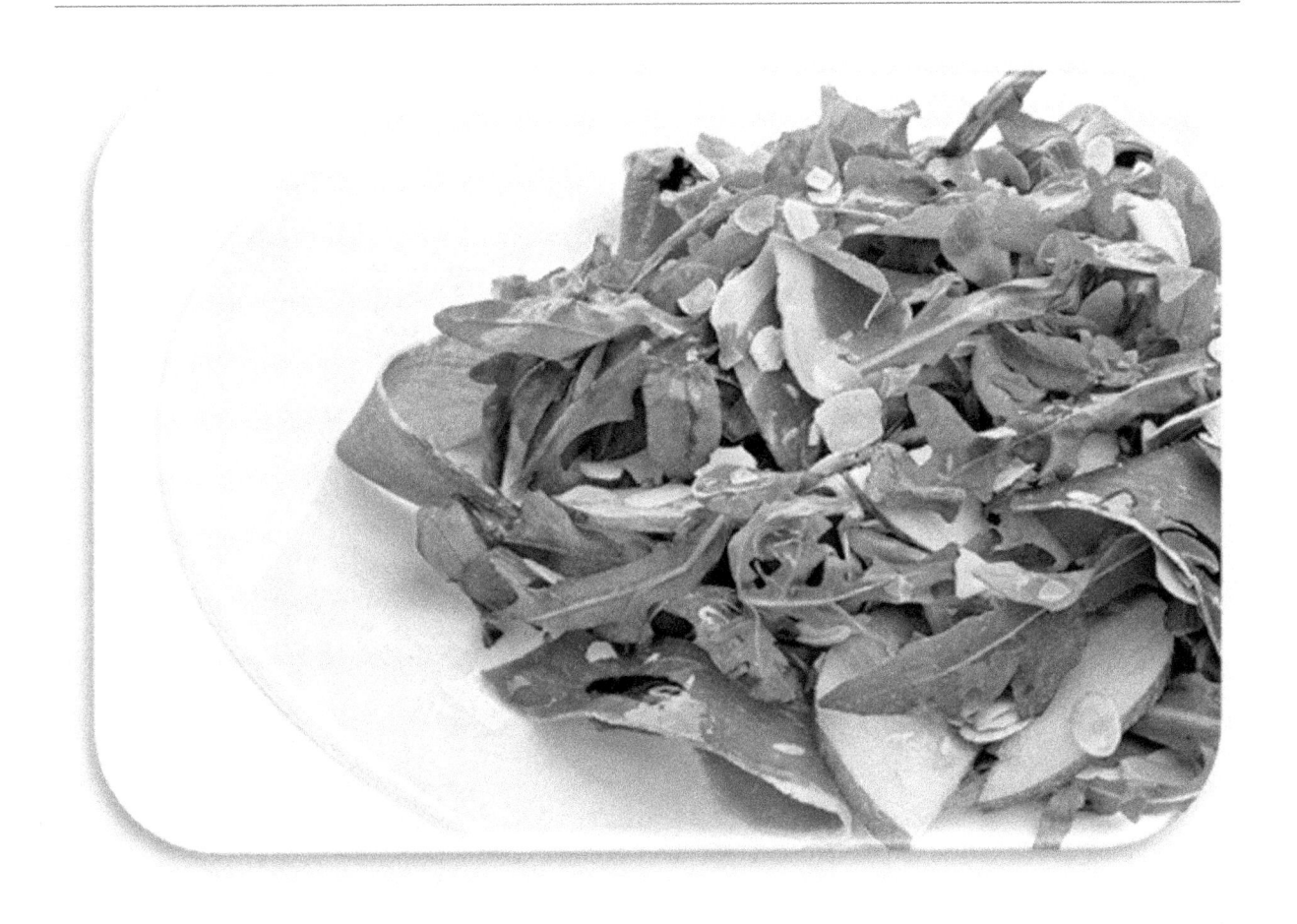

CARBS: 9.7 g | FAT: 12 g | PROTEIN: 8.6 g | CALORIES: 179

INGREDIENTS

- 3 oz bacon
- 1 pear, sliced
- 1 cup cherry tomatoes, halved
- 1 bell pepper, sliced
- 5 oz arugula, rinsed
- ¼ cup Parmesan, shredded
- 2 Tbsp pine nuts
- Olive oil for frying

DIRECTIONS

1. Arrange arugula at the bottom of a salad bowl and place tomatoes on it.
2. In a pan preheated with some olive oil add bacon, pepper and pear slices. Cook until the bacon pieces are crisp and the pear is more transparent.
3. Add bacon slices, pear and bell pepper to the salad bowl.
4. Sprinkle with Parmesan and pine nuts. Mix well.

NO BREAD BTL

SERVINGS: 1 | PREP TIME: 10 min. | COOK TIME: 10 min.

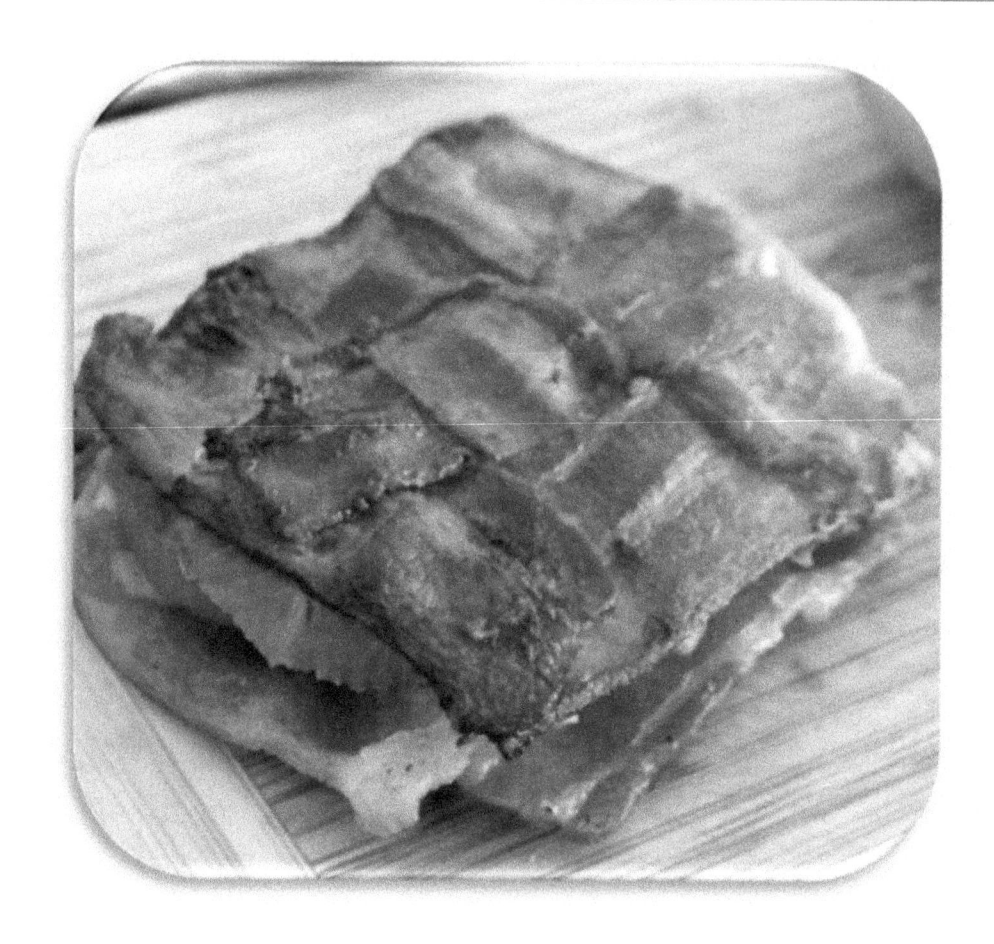

CARBS: 4 g | FAT: 52 g | PROTEIN: 17 g | CALORIES: 563

INGREDIENTS

- *6 slices bacon, sliced in half lengthwise to make 12 slices of the same length.*
- *1 tomato, sliced*
- *lettuce leaves*
- *Salt and pepper to taste*

DIRECTIONS

1. Make a basket weave with 3 parallel slices and 3 slices at right angles to these
2. Repeat to make another "basket".
3. Cook under a preheated broiler until the bacon starts to become crisp.
4. To serve add tomato slices and lettuce leaves between the two bacon "toasts".

AVOCADO RECIPES

AVOCADO AND SHRIMP SALAD

SERVINGS: 2 | PREP TIME: 15 min. | COOK TIME: 7 min.

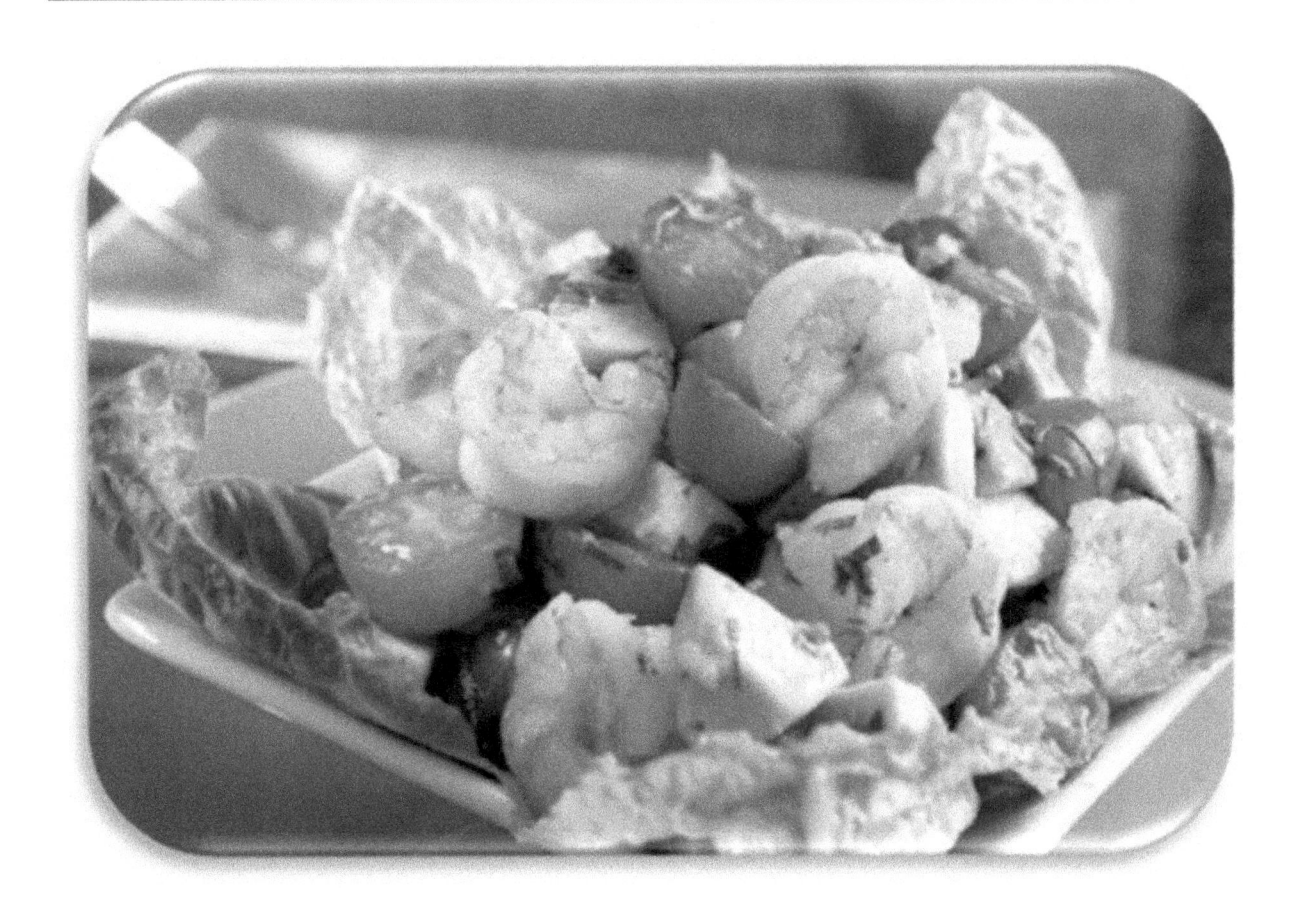

CARBS: 8.9 g | FAT: 18.5 g | PROTEIN: 38.6 g | CALORIES: 350

INGREDIENTS

- ½ avocado, peeled, sliced
- 4 cherry tomatoes. halved
- 20 shrimp, cooked, cooled
- 6 lettuce leaves, torn
- Lemon juice to taste
- Salt and pepper to taste
- 2 Tbsp Thousand Island Dressing

DIRECTIONS

1. Drizzle the sliced avocado with lemon juice, add tomatoes and lettuce leaves.
2. Add the cooked shrimp and dress the salad.

AVOCADO AND CUCUMBER SALAD

SERVINGS: 4 | PREP TIME: 10 min. | COOK TIME: 10 min.

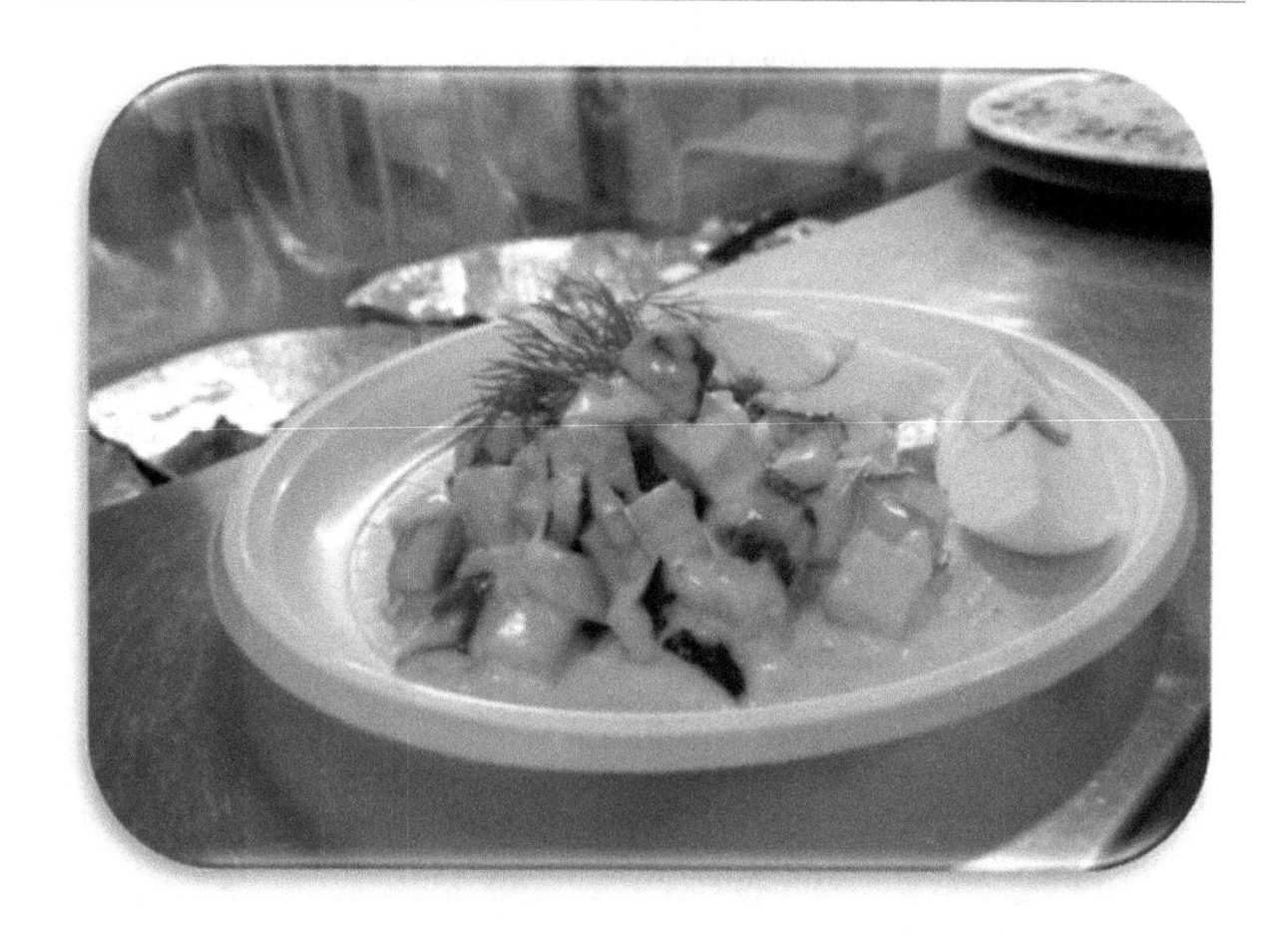

CARBS: 9.2 g | FAT: 19.5 g | PROTEIN: 7.7 g | CALORIES: 238

INGREDIENTS

- 1 avocado, peeled, pitted, cubed
- 2 cucumbers, cubed
- 3 eggs, hard-boiled. chopped
- Light mayonnaise for dressing
- Salt and pepper to taste

DIRECTIONS

1. Combine all ingredients and dress with mayonnaise.
2. Season with salt and pepper to taste and mix well.

AVOCADO SALSA

SERVINGS: 6 | PREP TIME: 10 min. | COOK TIME: 0 min.

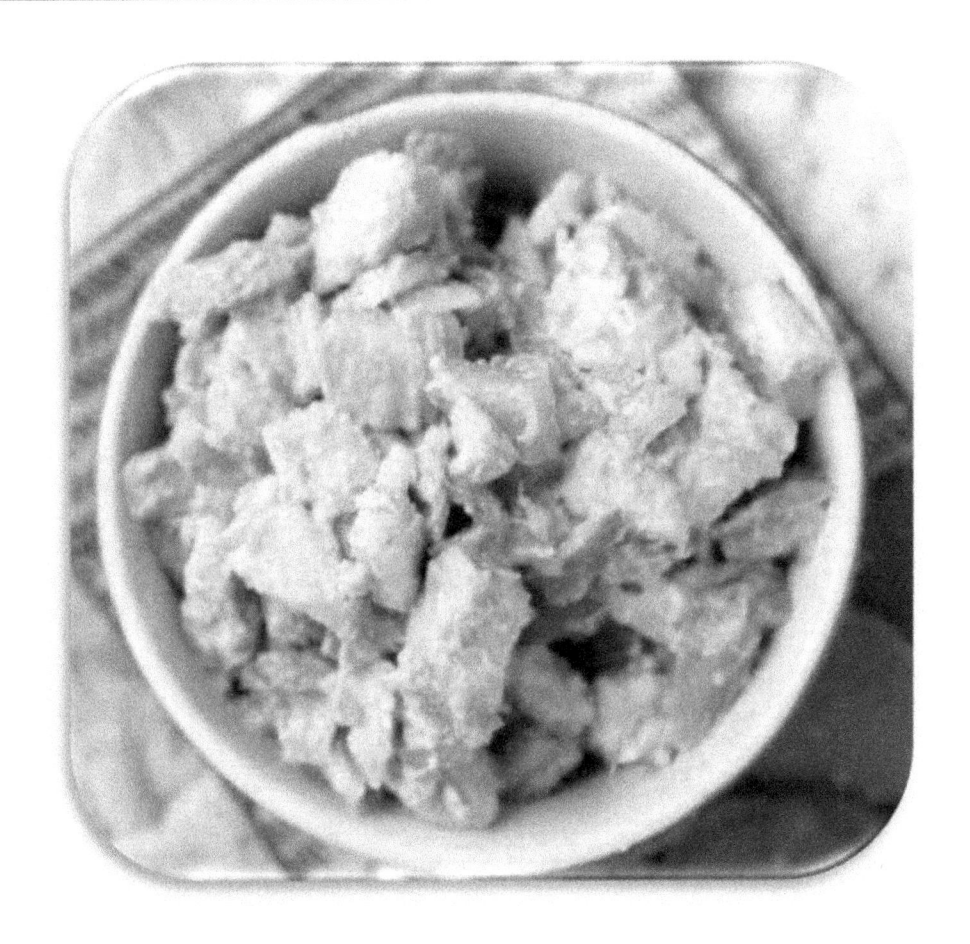

CARBS: 12 g | FAT: 14 g | PROTEIN: 2 g | CALORIES: 178

INGREDIENTS

- *4 avocados, peeled, pitted, diced*
- *2 tomatoes, diced*
- *1 red onion, diced*
- *1 fresh chili, diced*
- *1 lemon, juiced*

DIRECTIONS

1. Combine all ingredients and drizzle with lemon juice.
2. Season with salt and pepper to taste and mix well.

AVOCADO SALAD

SERVINGS: 4 | PREP TIME: 10 min. | COOK TIME: 0 min.

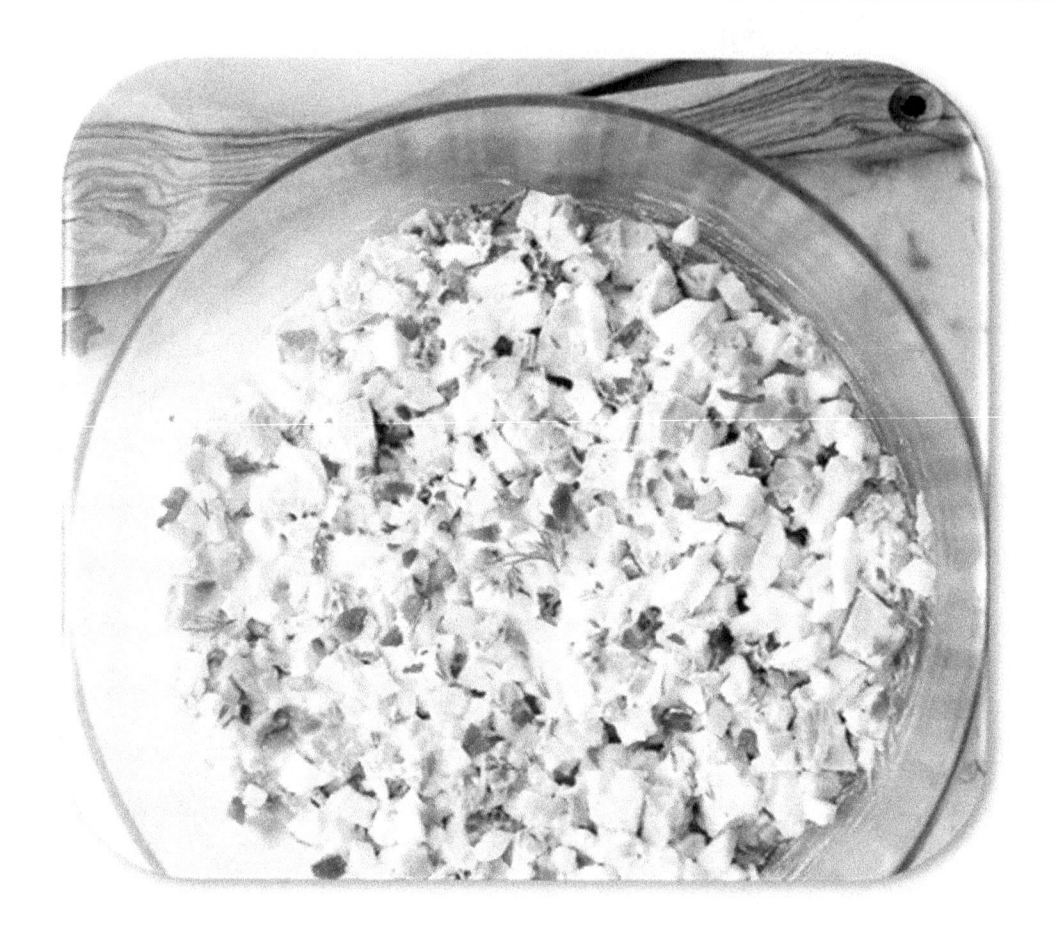

CARBS: 8 g | FAT: 21 g | PROTEIN: 11 g | CALORIES: 269

INGREDIENTS

- 1 avocado, peeled, pitted, diced
- 4 eggs, hard-boiled, minced
- 2 green onions, minced
- 4 bacon slices, cooked
- 1 lime, juiced
- 1 Tbsp sour cream
- ¼ cup plain yogurt
- 1 Tbsp fresh dill, minced
- Salt and pepper to taste

DIRECTIONS

1. In a salad bowl, combine diced eggs, avocado, green onions, and bacon.
2. Make the dressing by whisking the yogurt with sour cream and lime juice, add dill, salt and pepper.
3. Dress the salad with the yogurt dressing.

AVOCADO SPRING ROLLS

SERVINGS: 2 | PREP TIME: 10 min. | COOK TIME: 5 min.

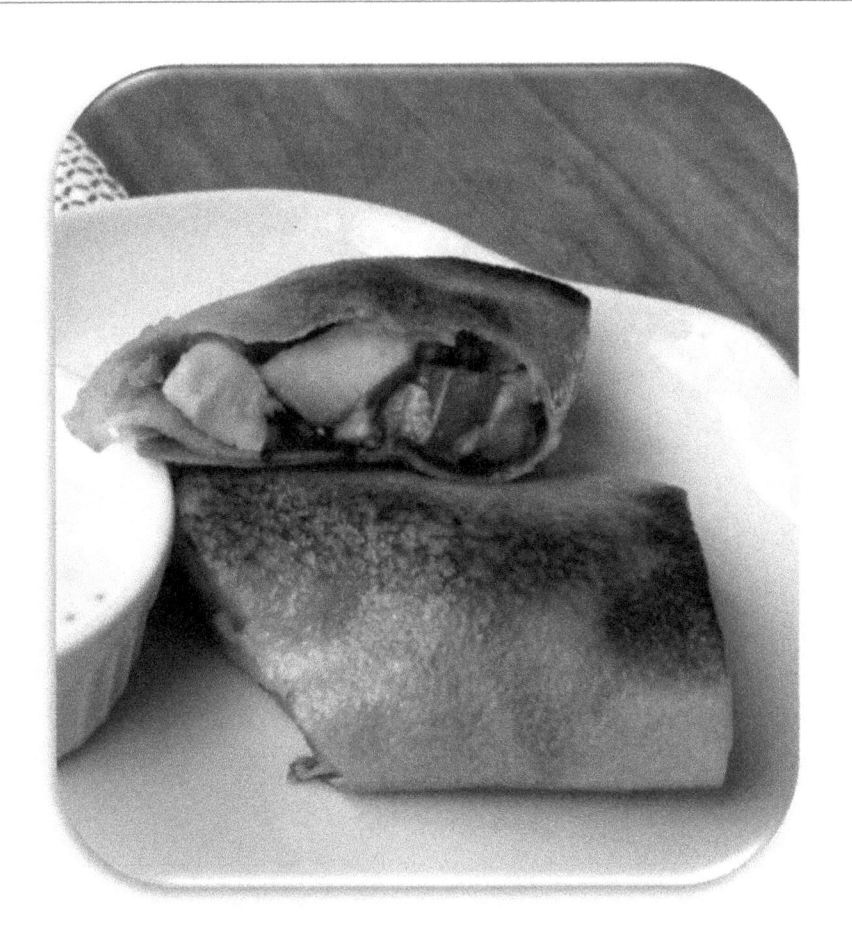

CARBS: 8 g | FAT: 14 g | PROTEIN: 5 g | CALORIES: 270

INGREDIENTS

- *1 avocado, peeled, pitted, diced*
- *½ tomato, diced*
- *3 Tbsp red onion, diced*
- *2 Tbsp cilantro leaves, chopped*
- *2 Keto/Paleo wraps*
- *1 Tbsp coconut oil*
- *½ lime, juiced*
- *Salt and pepper to taste*

DIRECTIONS

1. Combine avocado tomato, onions, cilantro leaves, salt and pepper and drizzle with lime juice.
2. Lay out keto wraps and divide the avocado mixture between the wraps.
3. Fold the paleo wrap inwards on two parallel sides, then roll until mixture is completely covered.
4. Fry in a pan preheated with oil on both sides (about 30 seconds each).

AVOCADO BOWL

SERVINGS: 2 | **PREP TIME:** 10 min. | **COOK TIME:** 5 min.

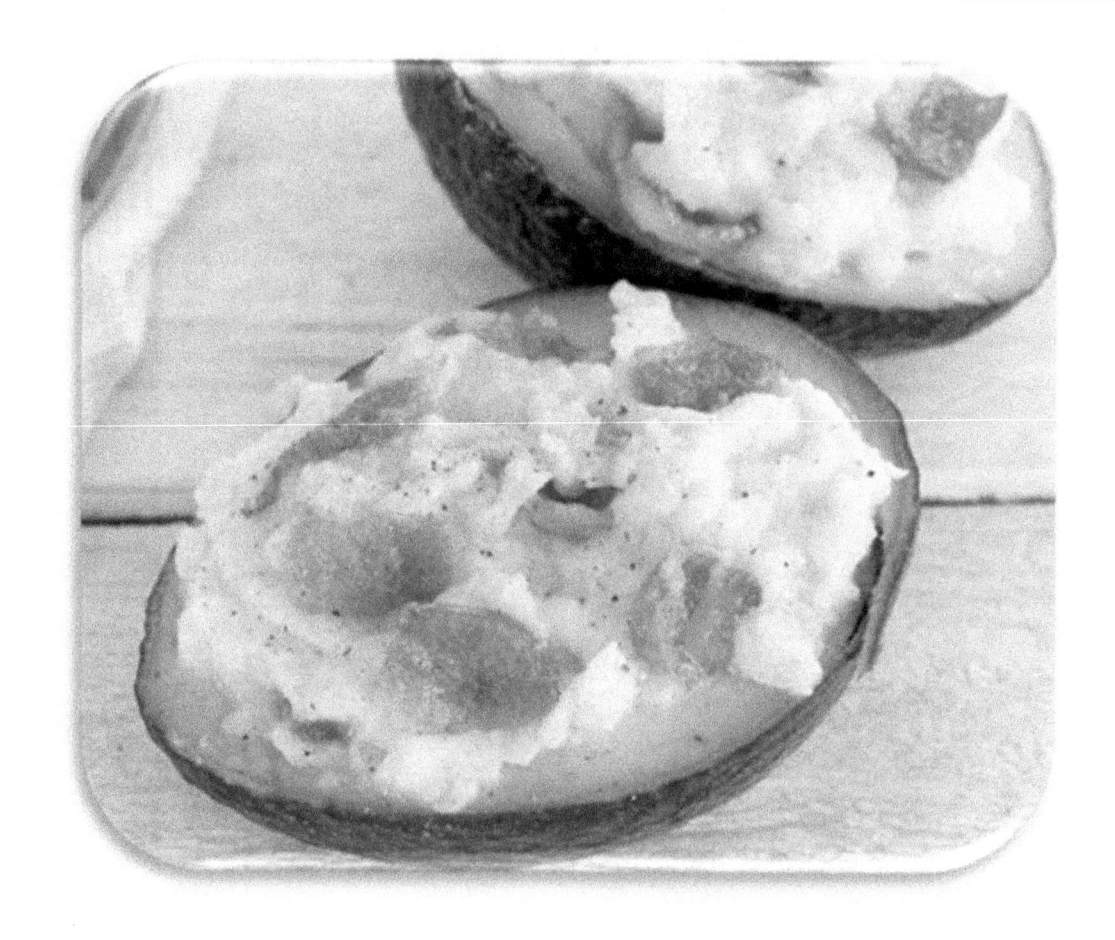

CARBS: 11 g | **FAT:** 40 g | **PROTEIN:** 25 g | **CALORIES:** 500

INGREDIENTS

- *1 avocado, pitted, flesh scooped out (1/2 inch left on shells)*
- *3 eggs, beaten with salt and pepper*
- *6 bacon slices, cut into pieces*
- *1 Tbsp butter*
- *Salt and pepper to taste*

DIRECTIONS

1. Heat butter in a saucepan and add bacon pieces to one side of a pan.
2. Add eggs to the other side of the pan, stirring to scramble.
3. Cook for 5 minutes and remove from heat.
4. Mix eggs with bacon and fill the avocado halves.

AVOCADO CASSEROLE

SERVINGS: 6 | PREP TIME: 15 min. | COOK TIME: 30 min.

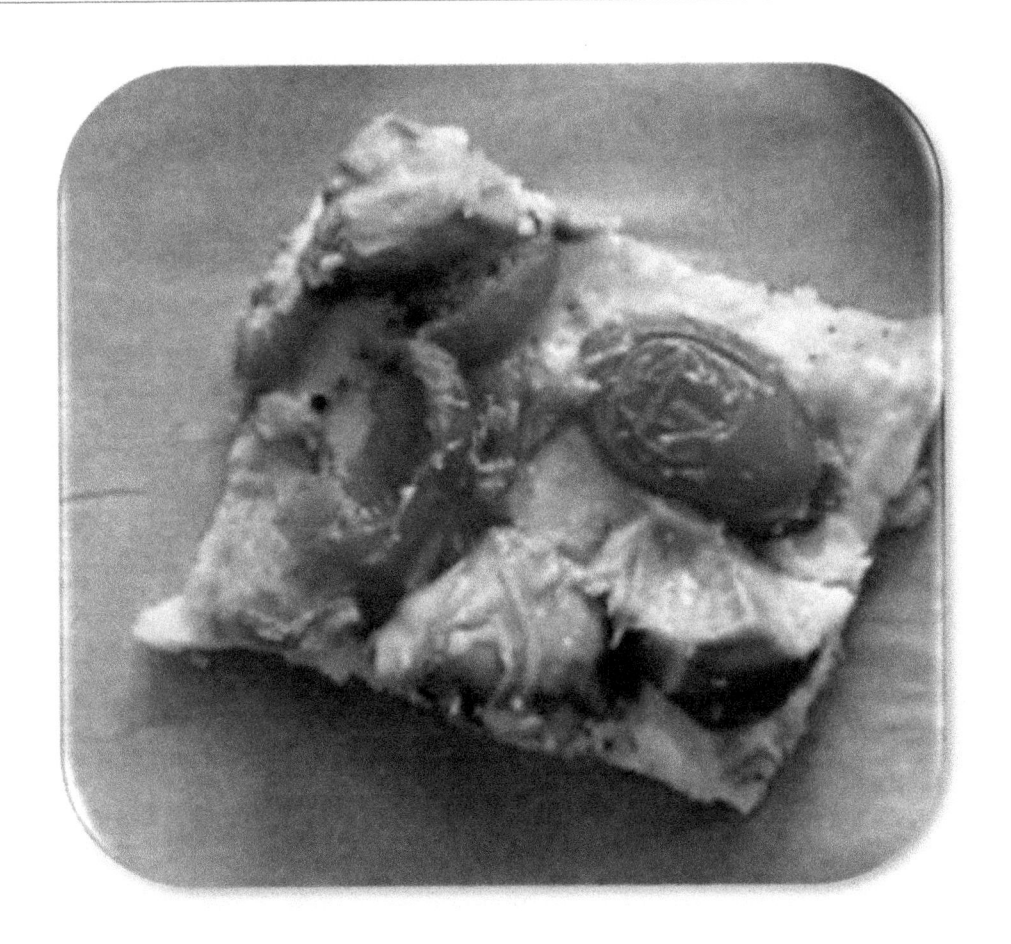

CARBS: 4.4 g | FAT: 26.4 g | PROTEIN: 20.4 g | CALORIES: 335

INGREDIENTS

- 1 avocado, peeled, pitted, diced
- 10 slices bacon, cooked
- 1 cup cherry tomatoes, halved
- 1 cup Cheddar, shredded
- 5 eggs
- ¼ cup keto friendly milk
- Salt and pepper to taste

DIRECTIONS

1. Layer bacon slices on a sprayed baking pan. Add tomatoes and avocado.
2. Beat eggs and milk together and pour the mixture over the bacon and avocado. Season with salt and pepper.
3. Sprinkle the cheese.
4. Bake for 30 minutes at 350°F.

AVOCADO FETA DIP

SERVINGS: 1 ¼ cup | **PREP TIME:** 2 min. | **COOK TIME:** 0 min.

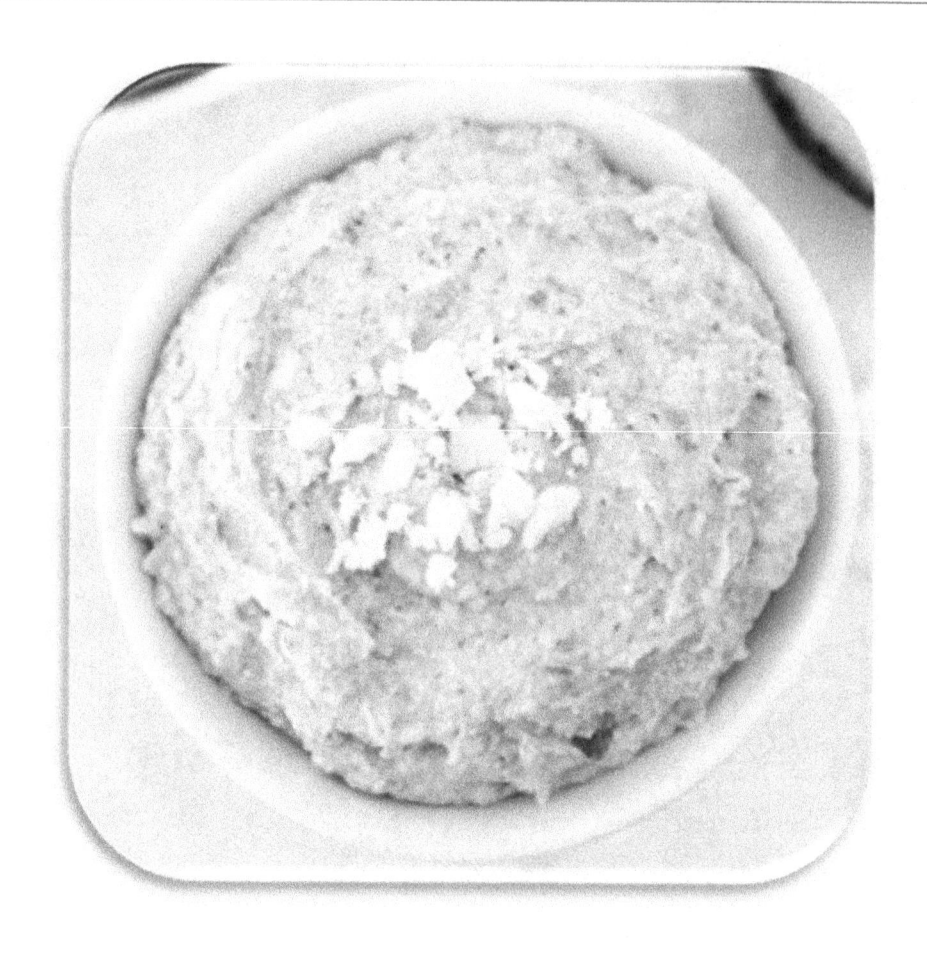

CARBS: 11 g | **FAT:** 17.4 g | **PROTEIN:** 4.9 g | **CALORIES:** 206

INGREDIENTS

- 2 avocados, peeled, pitted, diced
- ½ cup feta cheese
- ¼ cup onions, diced
- 1/3 cup cilantro, chopped
- 1 Tbsp jalapeño, minced
- 1 lime, juiced
- Salt and pepper to taste

DIRECTIONS

1. Add all ingredients to a food processor and pulse until smooth.
2. Serve with keto friendly crackers.

PROSCIUTTO-WRAPPED AVOCADO

SERVINGS: 8 | PREP TIME: 2 min. | COOK TIME: 0 min.

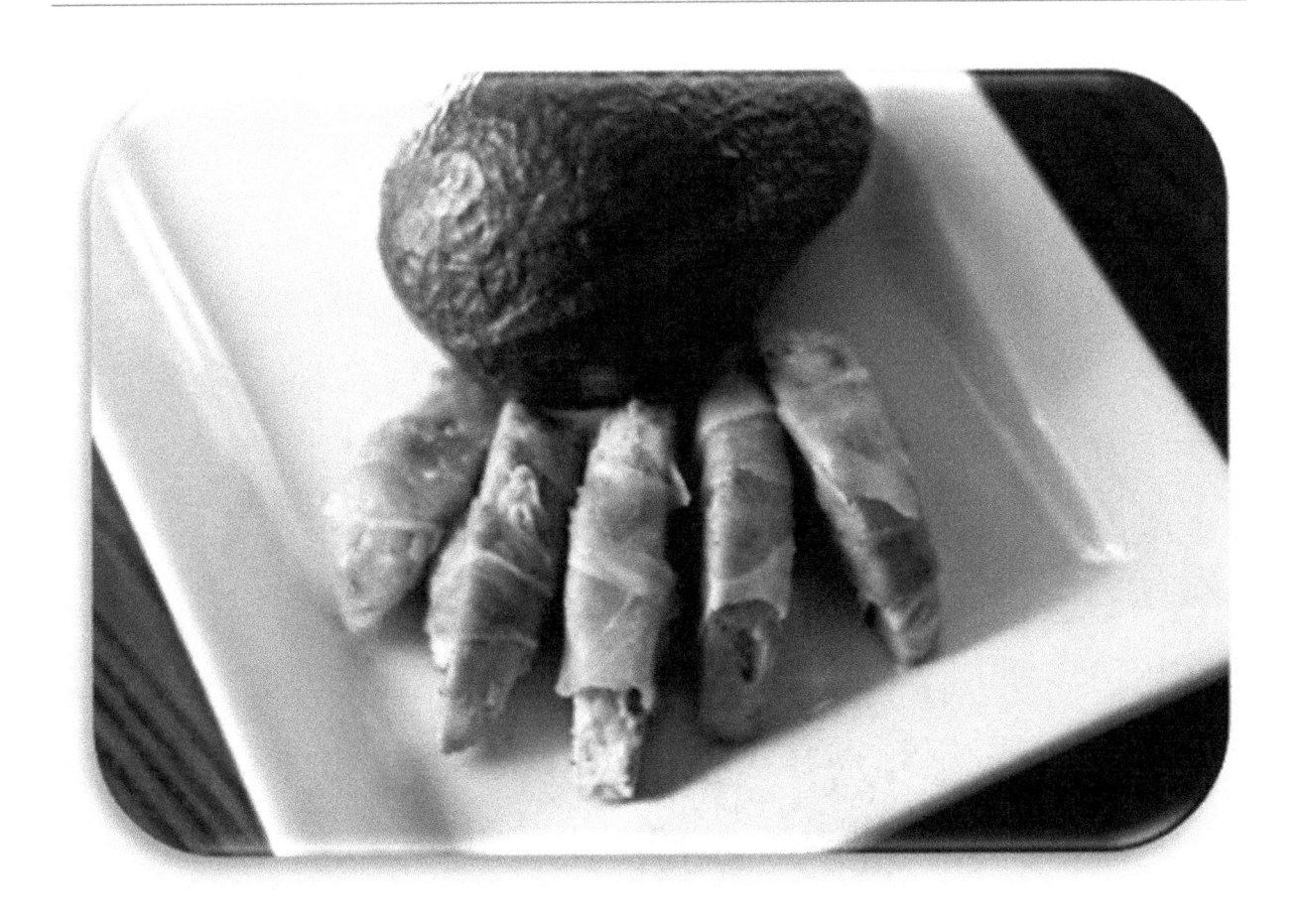

CARBS: 9 g | FAT: 21.6 g | PROTEIN: 4.2 g | CALORIES: 234

INGREDIENTS

- *4 avocados, peeled, pitted, halved*
- *1 oz prosciutto slices*
- *2 oz goat cheese*
- *1 Tbsp lime juice*
- *1 tsp chili powder*
- *Salt and pepper to taste*

DIRECTIONS

1. Cut each avocado half into 4–6 slices and sprinkle with lime juice.
2. Fill the center of each avocado slice with about ½ teaspoon goat cheese.
3. Season with salt, pepper and chili powder.
4. Wrap each avocado slice with a prosciutto slice or two, covering the goat cheese.

CUCUMBER ROLLS WITH AVOCADO

SERVINGS: 4 | PREP TIME: 5 min. | COOK TIME: 0 min.

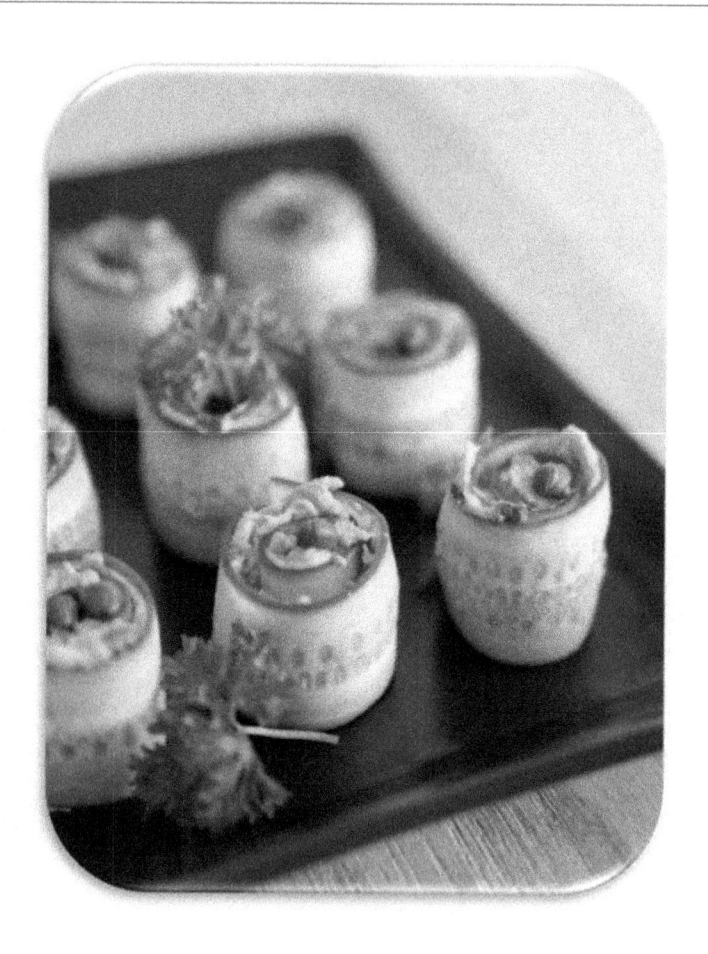

CARBS: 19 g | FAT: 20.3 g | PROTEIN: 4 g | CALORIES: 249

INGREDIENTS

- *3 avocados, peeled, pitted, mashed*
- *2 cucumbers, sliced thinly lengthwise*
- *¼ cup capers*
- *2 Tbsp lime juice*
- *¼ cup fresh parsley, minced*
- *⅛ cup fresh dill, minced*
- *Salt and pepper to taste*

DIRECTIONS

1. Lay out the cucumber slices.
2. Add lime juice to the avocado flesh and spread all the way across cucumber slices.
3. Roll up, making sure there is enough avocado spread at each end.
4. Garnish with minced parsley, dill and capers.

AVOCADO AND TUNA BROWN RICE

SERVINGS: 2 | PREP TIME: 5 min. | COOK TIME: 50 min.

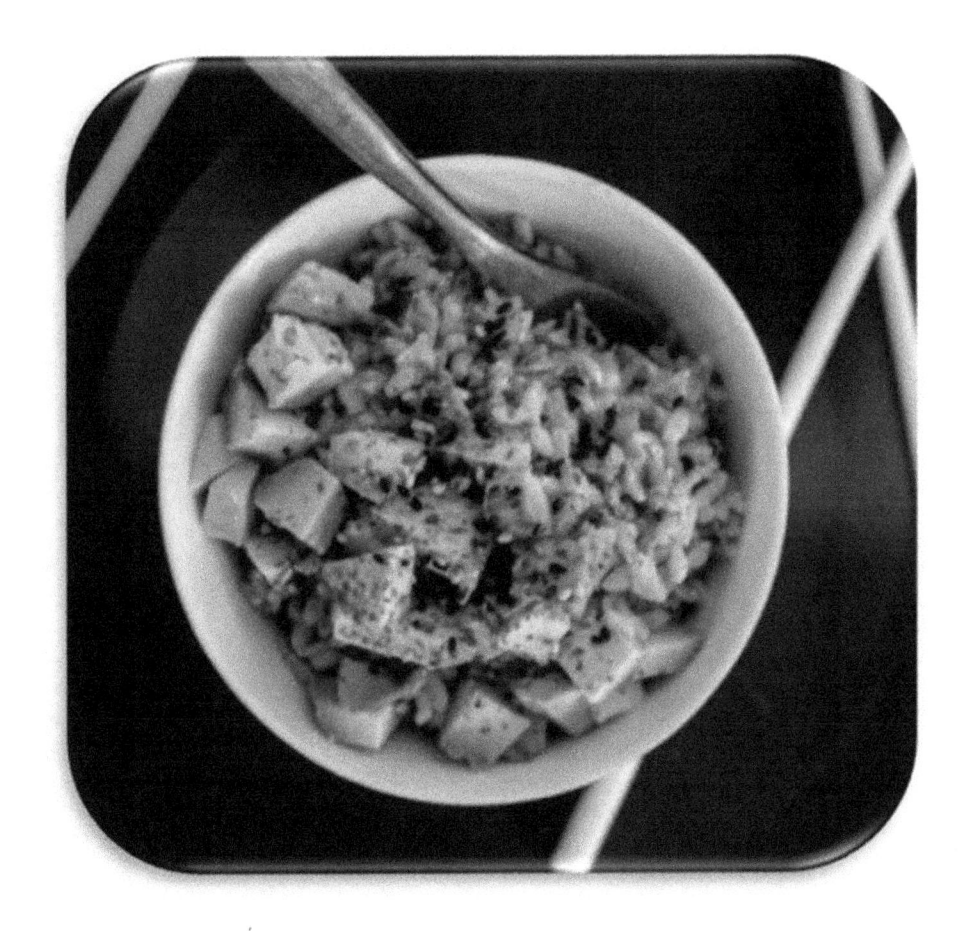

CARBS: 13.6 g | FAT: 17.1 g | PROTEIN: 63.5 g | CALORIES: 586

INGREDIENTS

- 1 avocado, peeled, pitted, cubed
- ½ cup brown rice, rinsed
- 1 can (5 oz) tuna, drained, flaked
- 2 eggs
- 1 tsp soy sauce
- ¼ tsp sesame oil
- ½ tsp rice vinegar
- Salt and pepper to taste
- 2 cups water

DIRECTIONS

1. Add 2 cups water to a saucepan; add rice, soy sauce and sesame oil.
2. Bring to boil. Let simmer on low, covered, for 25 minutes.
3. Drain the extra liquid from the rice and add tuna and rice vinegar to the rice, season with salt and pepper, stir
4. Cover and let stand for 10 minutes.
5. Fry the eggs, sunny side up.
6. Top the rice with avocado cubes.
7. Serve with fried eggs.

AVOCADO ICE CREAM

SERVINGS: 4 | PREP TIME: 7 h. 10 min. | COOK TIME: 0 min.

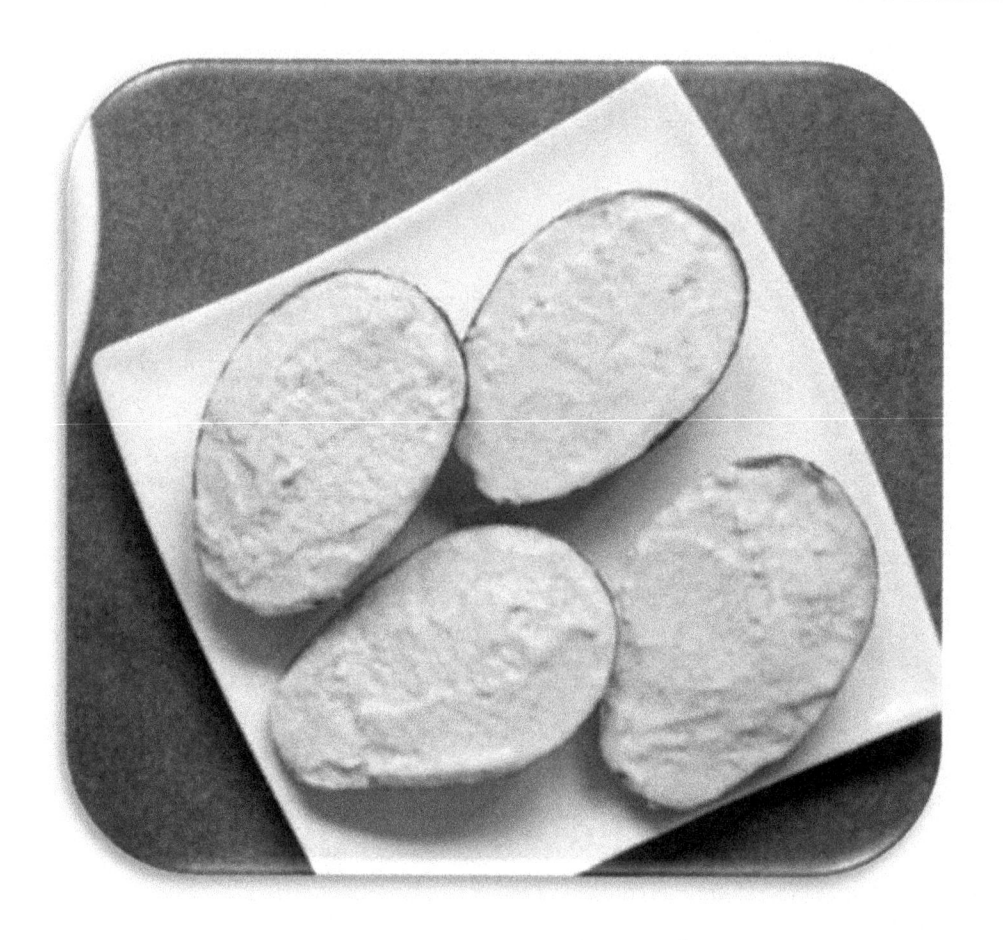

CARBS: 10.1 g | FAT: 31.4 g | PROTEIN: 2.8 g | CALORIES: 318

INGREDIENTS

- 2 avocados, halved, pitted, flesh scooped out
- 1 cup almond milk, unsweetened
- ⅓ cup erythritol
- ½ cup heavy cream

DIRECTIONS

1. Place the avocado shells into the freezer.
2. Blend together the avocado flesh, milk, erythritol, heavy cream and lemon juice.
3. Refrigerate for 5 hours.
4. If you have an ice cream maker process the mixture for 5–10 minutes in it and fill the avocado shells.
5. If not, beat the mixture with a hand mixer and fill the avocado shells.
6. Place the shells into the freezer for at least 2 hours.
7. Enjoy.

AVOCADO BARS

SERVINGS: 12 | PREP TIME: 2 h. | COOK TIME: 15 min.

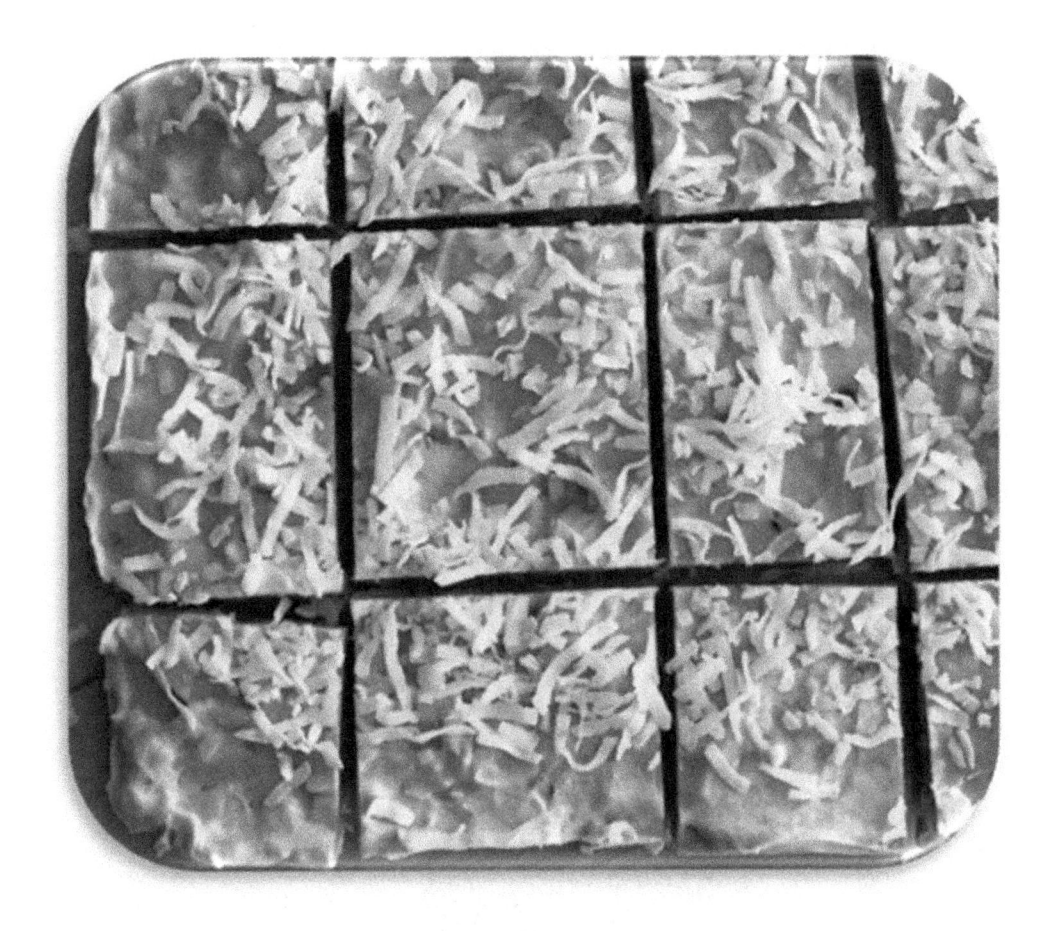

CARBS: 4.5 g | FAT: 13.9 g | PROTEIN: 1.7 g | CALORIES: 142

INGREDIENTS

- 2 avocados, peeled, pitted
- ½ cup heavy cream
- 3 Tbsp plain yogurt
- 1 Tbsp lemon juice
- ¼ cup Brazil nuts, chopped
- 2 Tbsp coconut, shredded, unsweetened
- 20 drops stevia

DIRECTIONS

1. In a food processor combine avocados, heavy cream, yogurt, lemon juice, and stevia. Blend.
2. In a separate bowl combine the blended mixture with coconut and Brazil nuts.
3. Line a baking sheet with parchment paper, spray with coconut oil and pour the mixture onto it.
4. Freeze for 2 hours.
5. Take the sheet out and slice into portions.

GREEN VEGETABLES RECIPES

CABBAGE PATTIES

SERVINGS: 6 | PREP TIME: 45 min. | COOK TIME: 15 min.

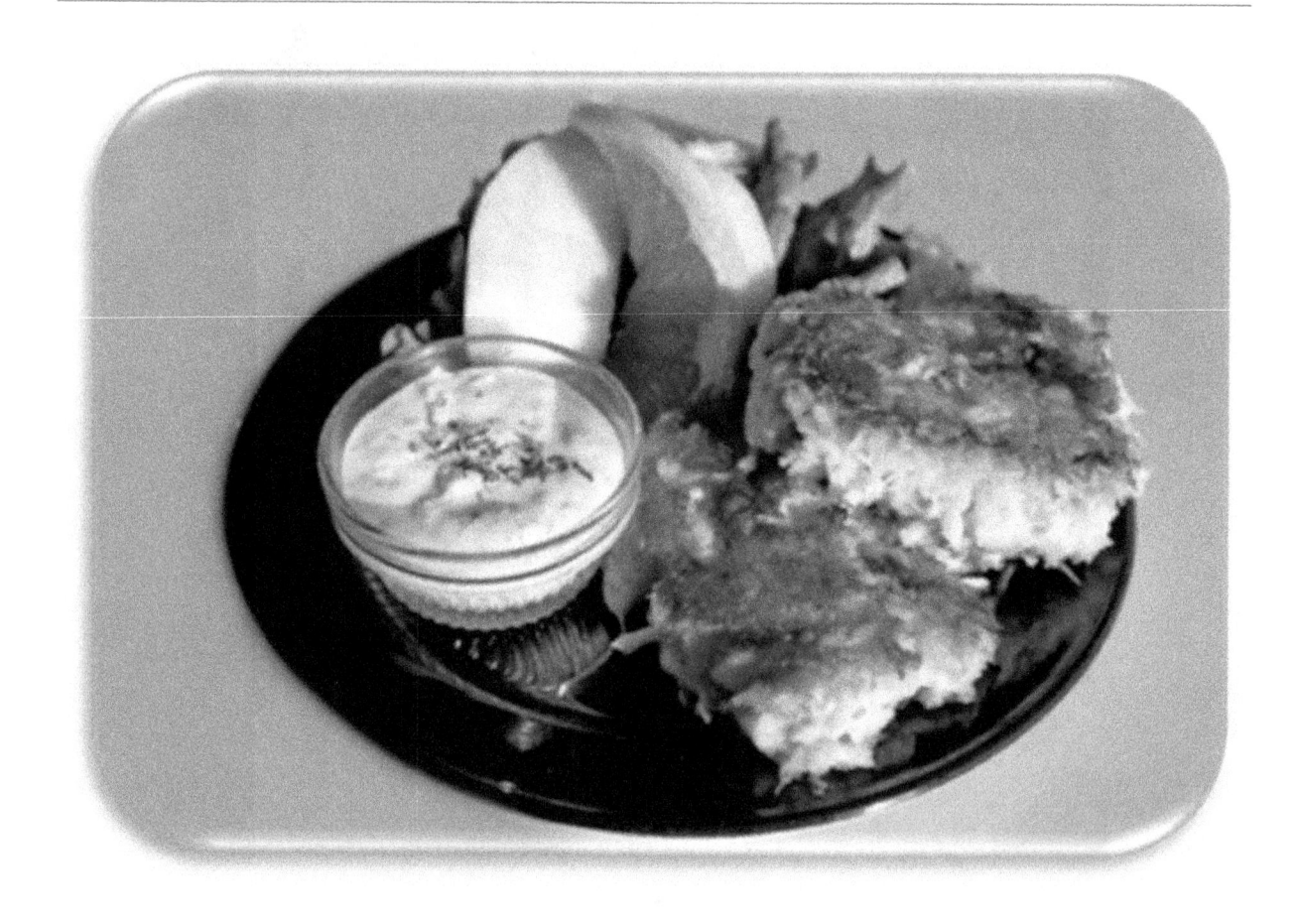

CARBS: 20 g | FAT: 5.7 g | PROTEIN: 7.8 g | CALORIES: 171

INGREDIENTS

- 2 lb 3 oz green cabbage, chopped
- 3 eggs
- ½–1 cup keto flour (almond / coconut)
- Olive oil for frying
- Salt and pepper to taste
- Sour cream to serve

DIRECTIONS

1. Add the chopped cabbage to a saucepan together with ½–1 cup water and bring to boil. Let simmer until the cabbage is soft.
2. Let cool and beat the eggs and flour, and season with salt and pepper. Mix well.
3. Shape the cabbage mixture into patties and fry in a frying pan preheated with olive oil.
4. Fry until golden. Serve with sour cream.

CABBAGE AND EGG SALAD

SERVINGS: 4 | PREP TIME: 15 min. | COOK TIME: 5 min.

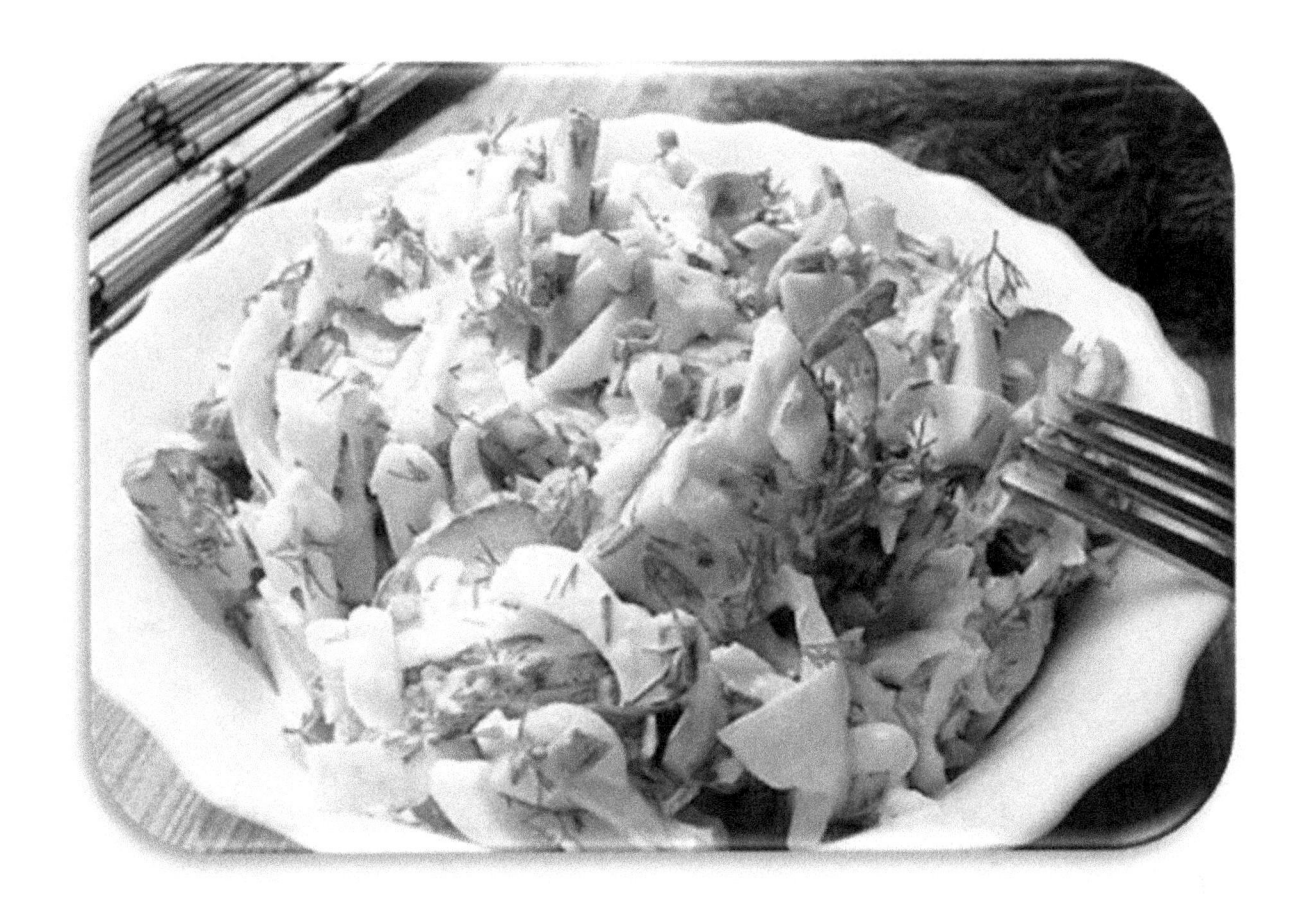

CARBS: 5 g | FAT: 13.1 g | PROTEIN: 4.1 g | CALORIES: 153

INGREDIENTS

- ½ head green cabbage, chopped
- 2 eggs, hard-boiled, chopped
- 1 tomato, chopped
- 1 cucumber, chopped
- 2 garlic cloves, minced
- 5-10 sprigs dill, minced
- 5-10 sprigs spring onions, minced
- Salt and pepper to taste
- Olive oil for dressing (about 3 Tbsp)

DIRECTIONS

1. Combine all chopped and minced ingredients and mix well. Dress with olive oil; season with salt and pepper.

KALE SALAD

SERVINGS: 4 | PREP TIME: 1 h. 3 min. | COOK TIME: 0 min.

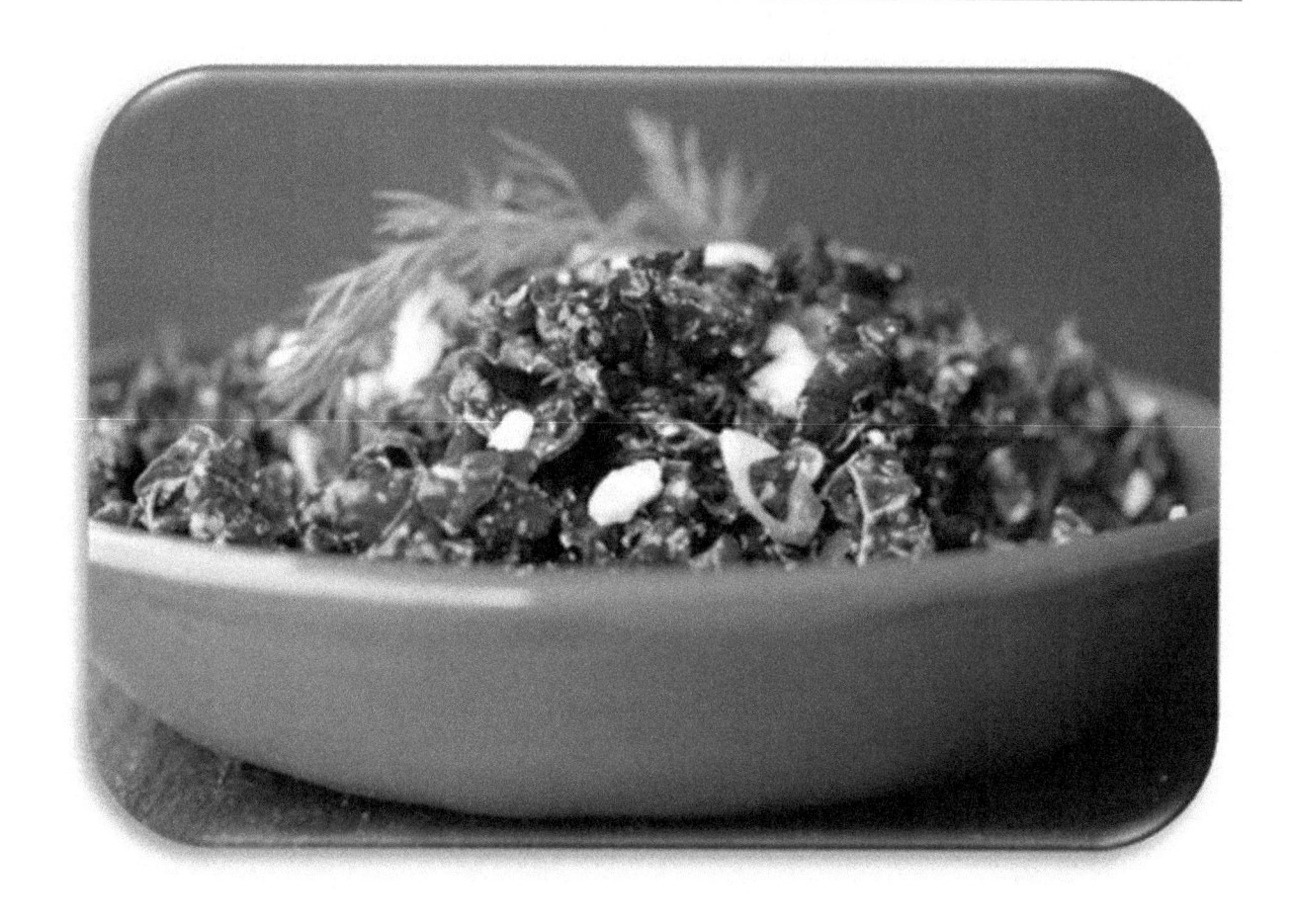

CARBS: 6 g | FAT: 20.9 g | PROTEIN: 4.4 g | CALORIES: 221

INGREDIENTS

- *4-5 oz kale, cut in strips*
- *1 shallot, sliced into rings*
- *1 garlic clove*
- *⅓ cup feta, crumbled*
- *⅓ cup pine nuts*
- *3 Tbsp olive oil*
- *1.5 Tbsp lemon juice*
- *Salt and pepper to taste*

DIRECTIONS

1. Add kale and shallots to a bowl.
2. Mix together olive oil, lemon juice and ½ tsp salt.
3. Dress kale and shallots with oil mixture and let stand for an hour.
4. Add feta, nuts, garlic and season with pepper to taste.

GREEN EASTERN SALAD

SERVINGS: 4 | PREP TIME: 5 min. | COOK TIME: 0 min.

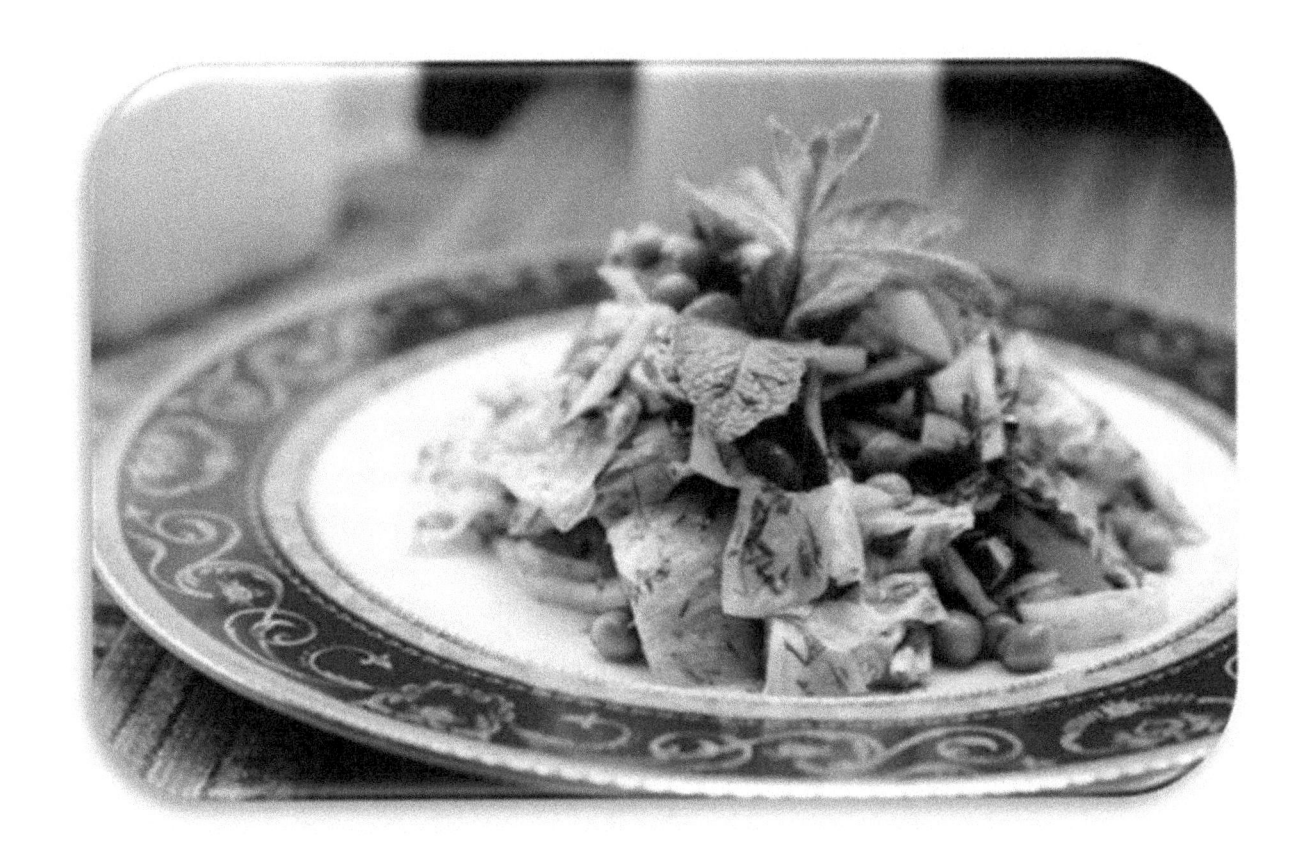

CARBS: 1.9 g | FAT: 7.1 g | PROTEIN: 1.1 g | CALORIES: 77

INGREDIENTS

- ¾ cup iceberg lettuce, torn
- ¼ cup cucumber, cut into straws
- ¼ cup green peas
- 5-10 sprigs fresh dill and fresh parsley, minced
- 1 Tbsp fresh mint, minced
- 1 Tbsp lemon juice
- 2 Tbsp olive oil
- Salt and pepper to taste

DIRECTIONS

1. Combine all ingredients in a salad bowl, season with salt and pepper. Dress with olive oil and lemon juice.

CHICKEN FILLETS BAKED WITH BROCCOLI

SERVINGS: 4 | PREP TIME: 7 min. | COOK TIME: 35 min.

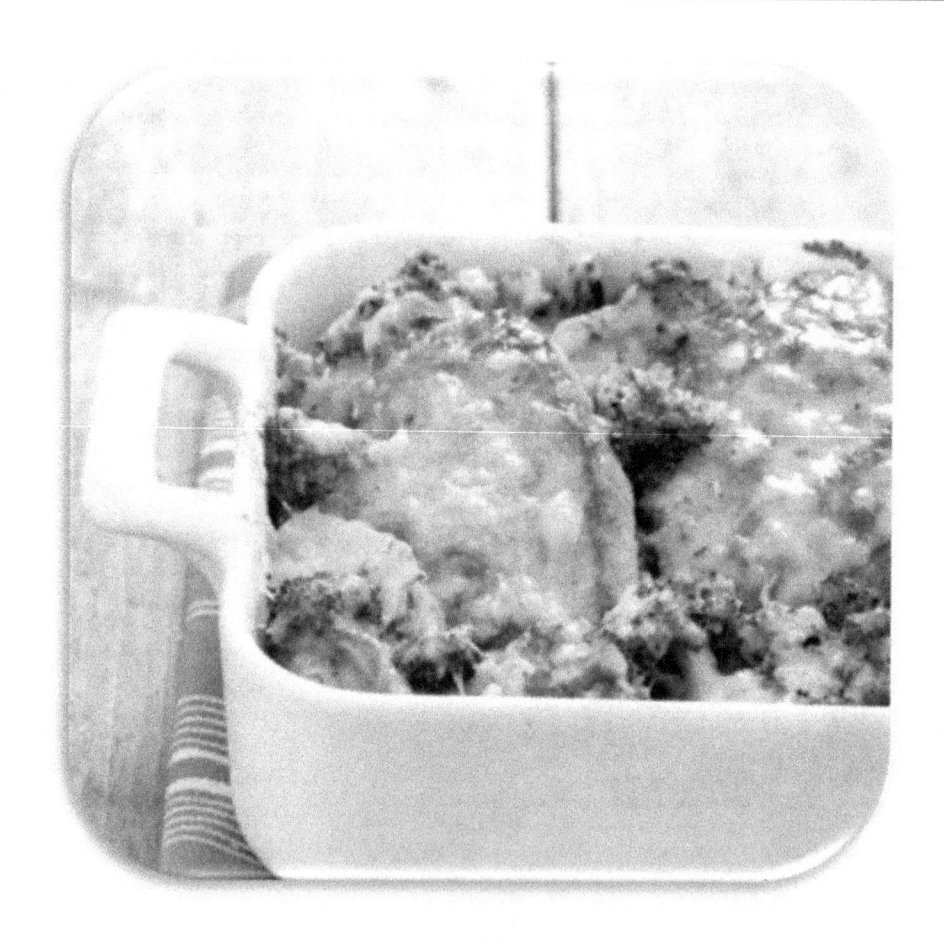

CARBS: 25 g | FAT: 43 g | PROTEIN: 42.4 g | CALORIES: 664

INGREDIENTS

- 4 chicken breast fillets, skinless
- 3 cups broccoli florets
- 1½ cups Parmesan, grated
- 4 Tbsp butter
- 1 onion, chopped
- 1 cup chicken stock
- ½ cup cream
- ½ cup dry sherry
- Salt and pepper to taste

DIRECTIONS

1. Season the fillets with salt and pepper. Heat 1 Tbsp butter in a frying pan and add chicken fillets. Fry for about 3 minutes on each side.
2. Remove the chicken, add 3 Tbsp butter to the same pan, and cook onions for 3 minutes until golden.
3. Add chicken stock, cream and sherry to the pan and bring to a boil. Let simmer for about 3 minutes.
4. Transfer the chicken back to the pan and cook, covered, for 15, minutes over medium heat.
5. Transfer the chicken with the sauce to an oven proof dish. Add broccoli florets, sprinkle with 1 cup Parmesan. Season with salt and pepper.
6. Transfer the dish to the oven, sprinkle with the remaining Parmesan and bake for 4 minutes at 356F.

BROCCOLI AND MUSHROOM QUICHE TITLE

SERVINGS: 6 | PREP TIME: 15 min. | COOK TIME: 20 min.

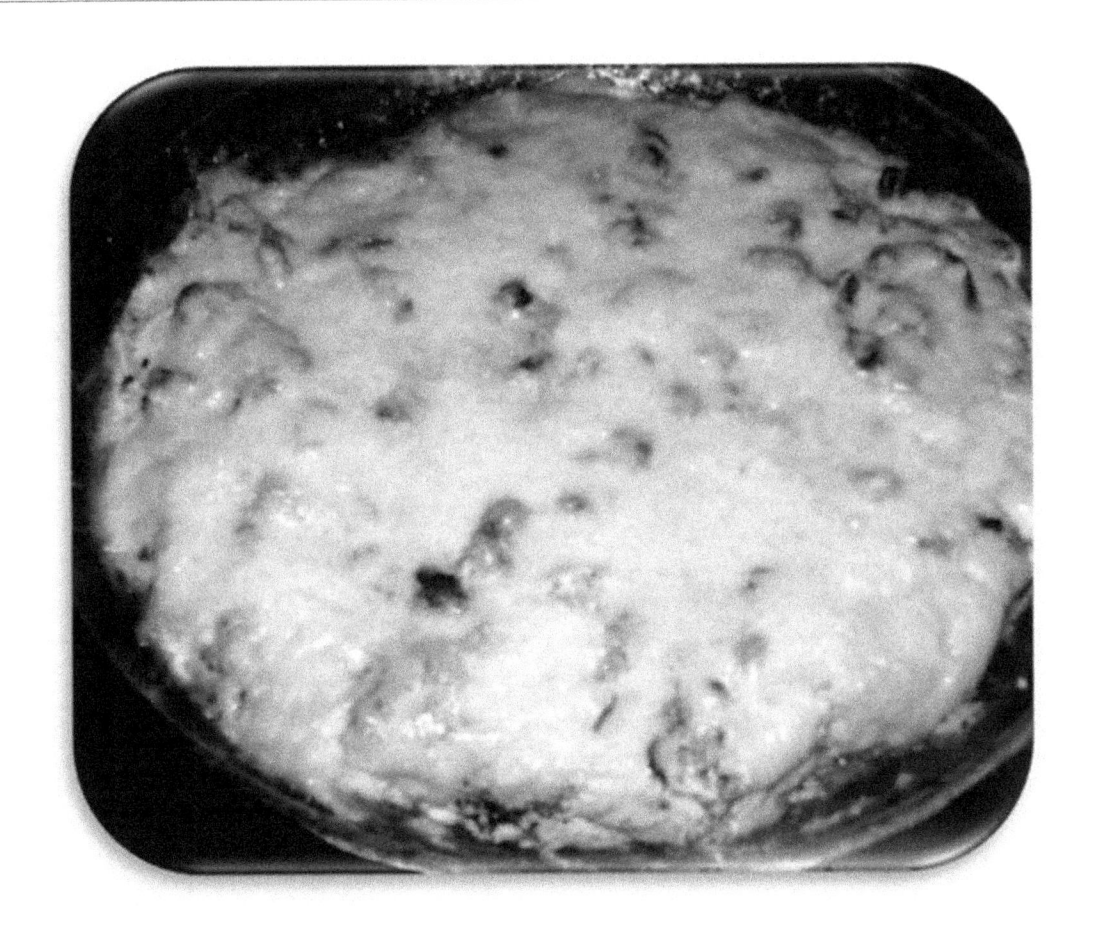

CARBS: 8.8 g | FAT: 44.2 g | PROTEIN: 21.2 g | CALORIES: 506

INGREDIENTS

- 3 cups broccoli florets, boiled, half-cooked (see instructions)
- 18 oz (4 cups) white mushrooms, rinsed, cleaned
- 4 eggs
- 1½ cups sour cream
- 1½ cups hard cheese, grated
- 1¾ sticks (7 oz) butter
- Salt and pepper to taste

DIRECTIONS

1. Heat the butter in a frying pan and cook the mushrooms for about 20 minutes over medium heat.
2. To make the broccoli half-cooked, drop the florets into boiling water and boil for 2 minutes.
3. In a bowl beat the eggs together with sour cream.
4. Transfer mushrooms and broccoli to an oven-proof dish and pour in the egg mixture. Season with salt and pepper.
5. Sprinkle with cheese.
6. Bake for 15–20 minutes at 356°F.

BROCCOLI IN ORANGE SAUCE

SERVINGS: 4 | PREP TIME: 5 min. | COOK TIME: 15 min.

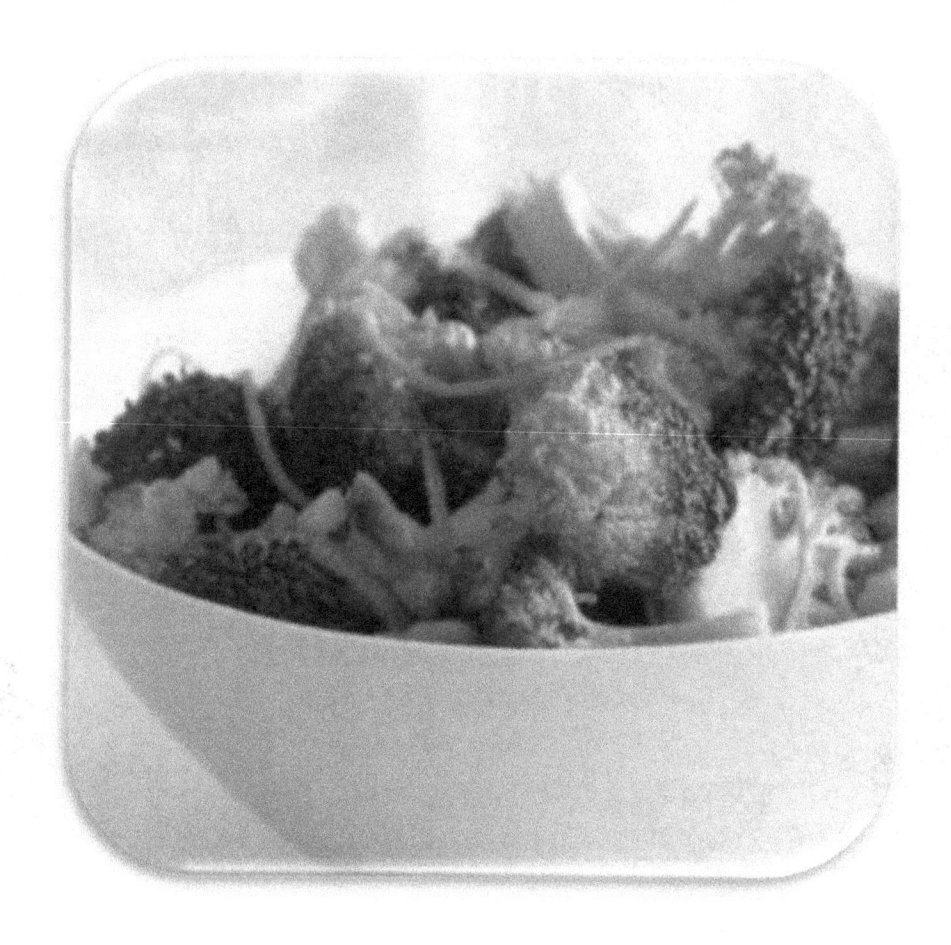

CARBS: 10 g | FAT: 10.4 g | PROTEIN: 5 g | CALORIES: 145

INGREDIENTS

- 5 cups broccoli florets
- 1 orange, peeled (zest saved)
- 1 Tbsp olive oil
- 1 Tbsp soy sauce
- ½ tsp fresh ginger, grated finely
- ⅓ cup walnuts, chopped
- Salt and pepper to taste

DIRECTIONS

1. Cut the orange zest into thin strips. Juice the orange and use only ¼ cup of squeezed juice.
2. Heat olive oil in a deep pan and add orange zest, walnuts and ginger. Fry, stirring, for 2 minutes.
3. Pour into the pan ¼ cup orange juice and the soy sauce. Add broccoli florets. Cook stirring until soft.

SPINACH WITH TOMATOES

SERVINGS: 4 | PREP TIME: 5 min. | COOK TIME: 15 min.

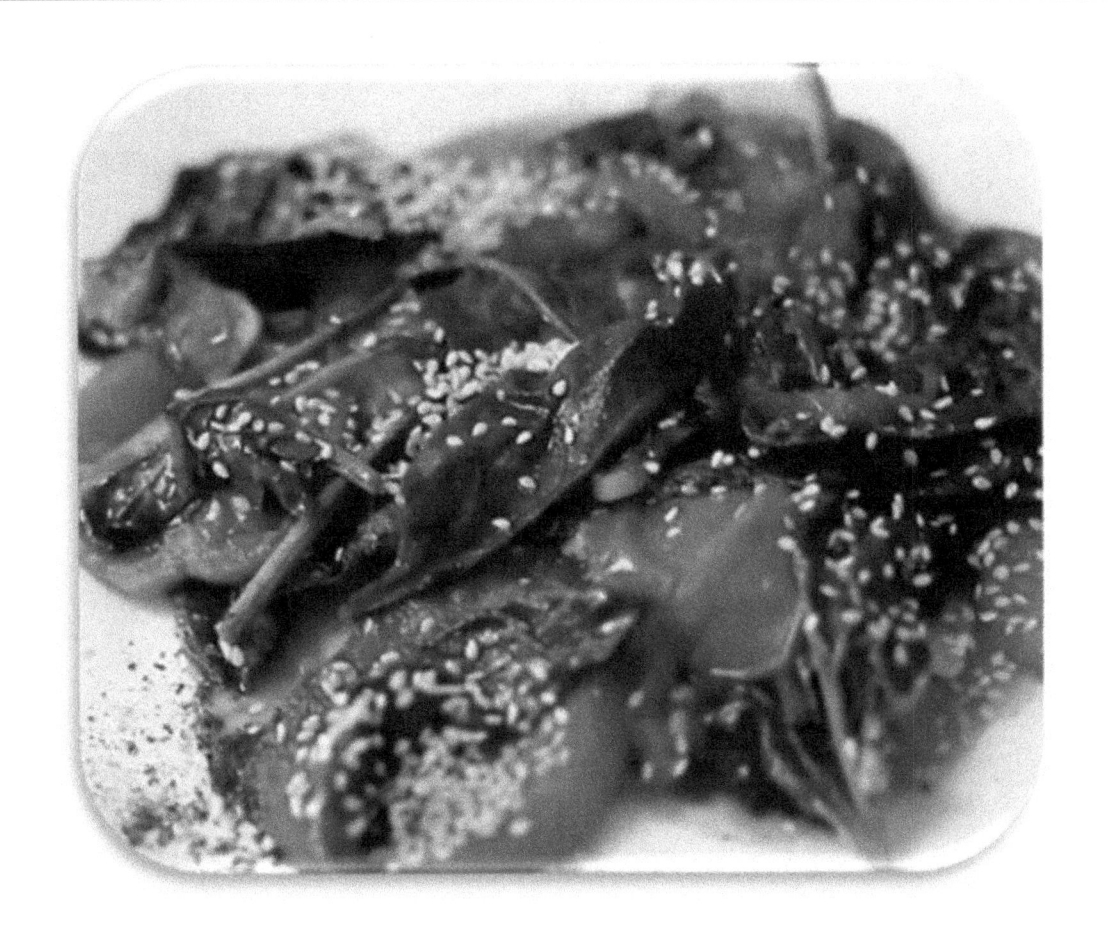

CARBS: 7 g | FAT: 1.6 g | PROTEIN: 3.6 g | CALORIES: 54

INGREDIENTS

- *2 cups spinach, stalks removed*
- *3 tomatoes, sliced in rounds*
- *2 garlic cloves, chopped in big chunks*
- *1 Tbsp sesame seeds*
- *Salt and pepper to taste*
- *Olive oil for frying*

DIRECTIONS

1. Add some olive oil to a frying pan and fry the tomato rounds for about a minute.
2. Add garlic cloves and spinach leaves.
3. Cook stirring occasionally until the leaves are soft.
4. Transfer to serving plates. Season with salt, pepper and sesame seeds.

SPINACH SALAD WITH TUNA

SERVINGS: 4 | PREP TIME: 5 min. | COOK TIME: 0 min.

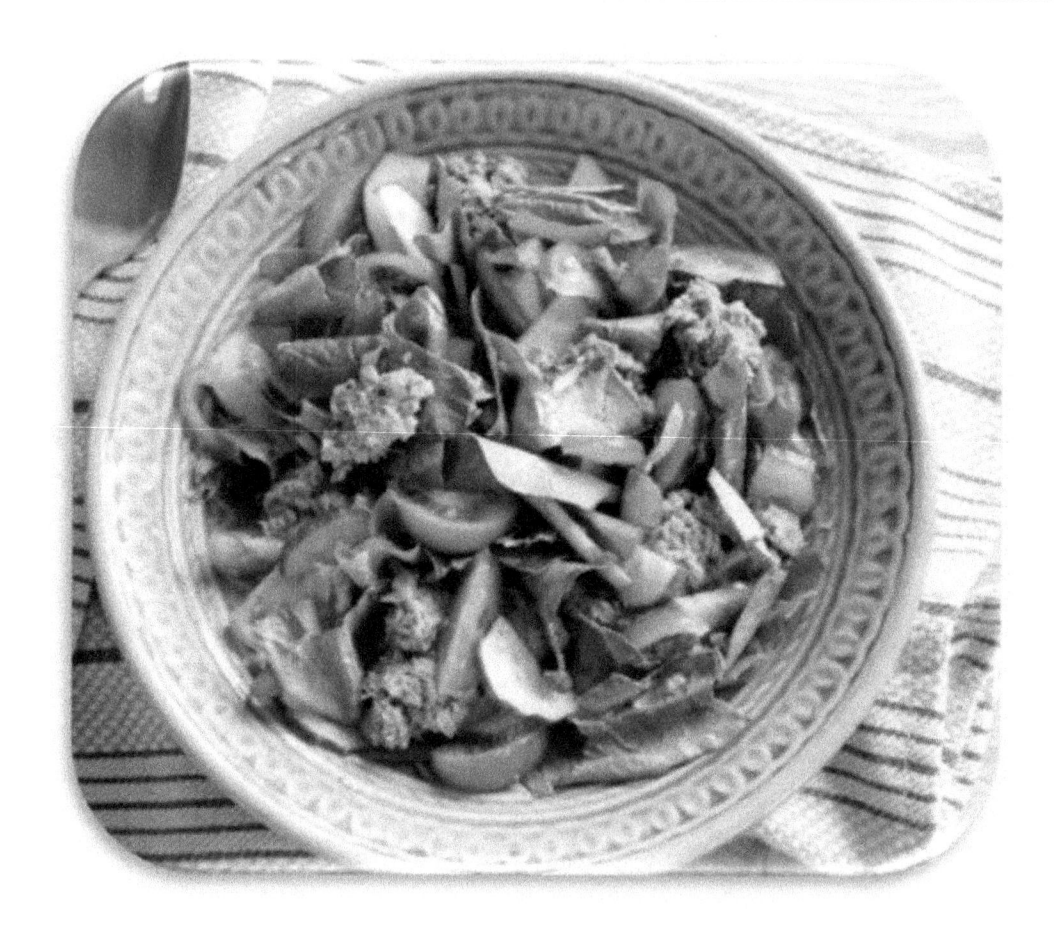

CARBS: 12.5 g | FAT: 11.5 g | PROTEIN: 6.2 g | CALORIES: 189

INGREDIENTS

- 4 cups spinach, rinsed, stalks removed, leaves torn
- 1 can (about 5–6 oz) tuna, chopped
- 3 tomatoes, sliced
- 1 cucumber, sliced
- 1 Tbsp lemon juice
- 3 Tbsp olive oil
- 1 tsp Dijon mustard
- Salt and pepper to taste

DIRECTIONS

1. Combine all ingredients in a salad bowl.
2. Prepare the dressing by mixing together olive oil, lemon juice and Dijon mustard.
3. Pour the dressing over the salad, mix well.

SPINACH ROLLS

SERVINGS: 4 | PREP TIME: 20 min. | COOK TIME: 30 min.

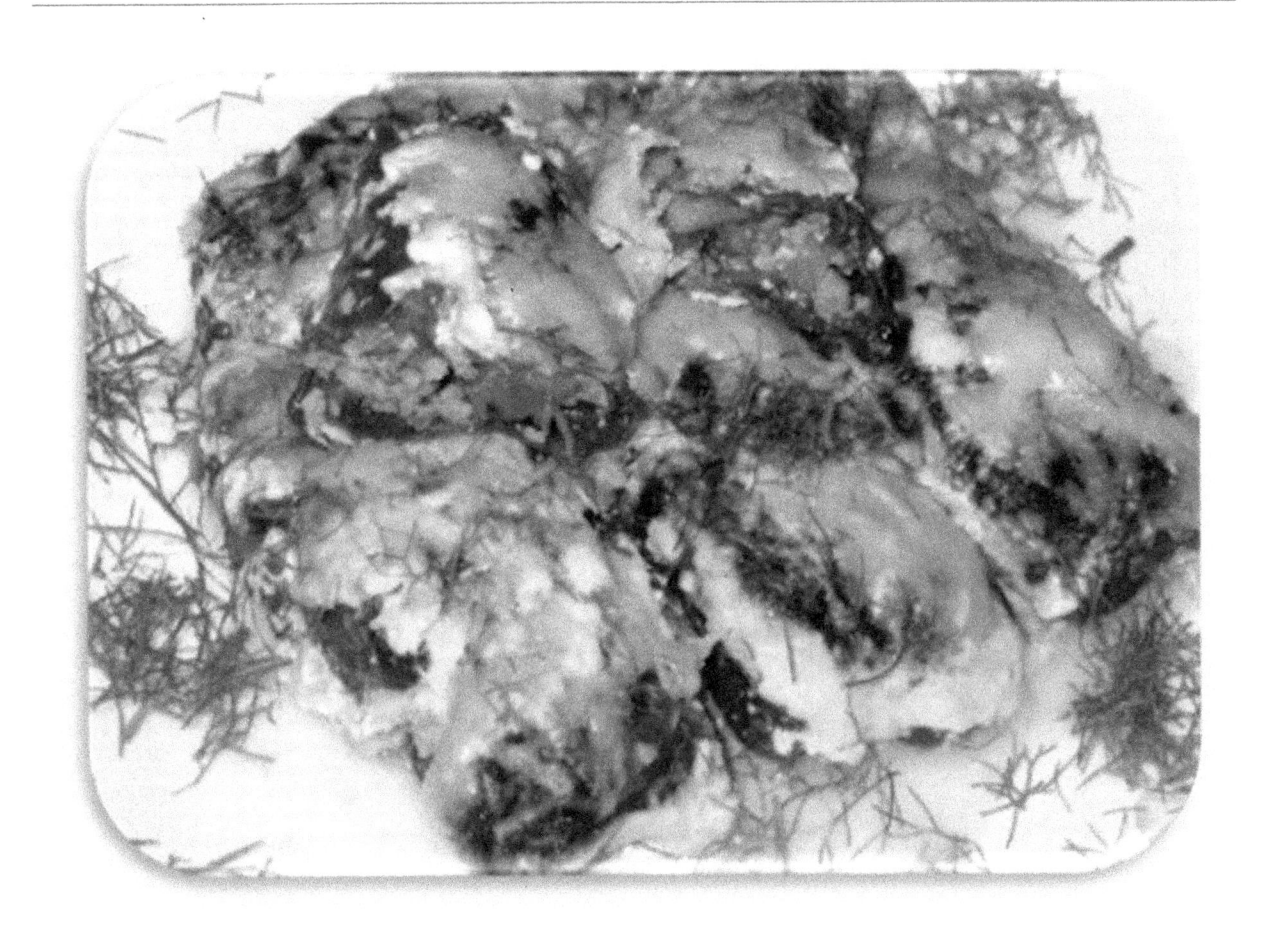

CARBS: 26 g | FAT: 49.9 g | PROTEIN: 53.5 g | CALORIES: 706

INGREDIENTS

- *20 large spinach leaves, rinsed*
- *1 lb ground meat to your liking (turkey/chicken/beef&pork)*
- *1 onion, minced*
- *1 tomato, cubed*
- *¼ green bell pepper, chopped*
- *2 Tbsp olive oil*
- *½ cup hard cheese*
- *1–2 cups sour cream*
- *Salt and red pepper to taste*
- *Olive oil for frying*

DIRECTIONS

1. Parboil the spinach leaves in boiling water for 3 minutes. Drain under cold water and dry.
2. Sauté onions in olive oil in a deep pan for 2 minutes, add green pepper.
3. Add ground meat and cook for 10 minutes.
4. Add tomato cubes and let simmer for 5 minutes.
5. Season with salt and pepper.
6. Place the meat filling in the center of each spinach leaf and roll the leaves, folding in the ends.
7. Arrange the spinach rolls in an oven proof pan, in one layer if possible. Season with red pepper.
8. Pour over the sour cream.
9. Bake for 20 minutes at 356°F.
10. Sprinkle with cheese and bake for 10 more minutes.

MOZZARELLA SPINACH

SERVINGS: 4 | PREP TIME: 20 min. | COOK TIME: 30 min.

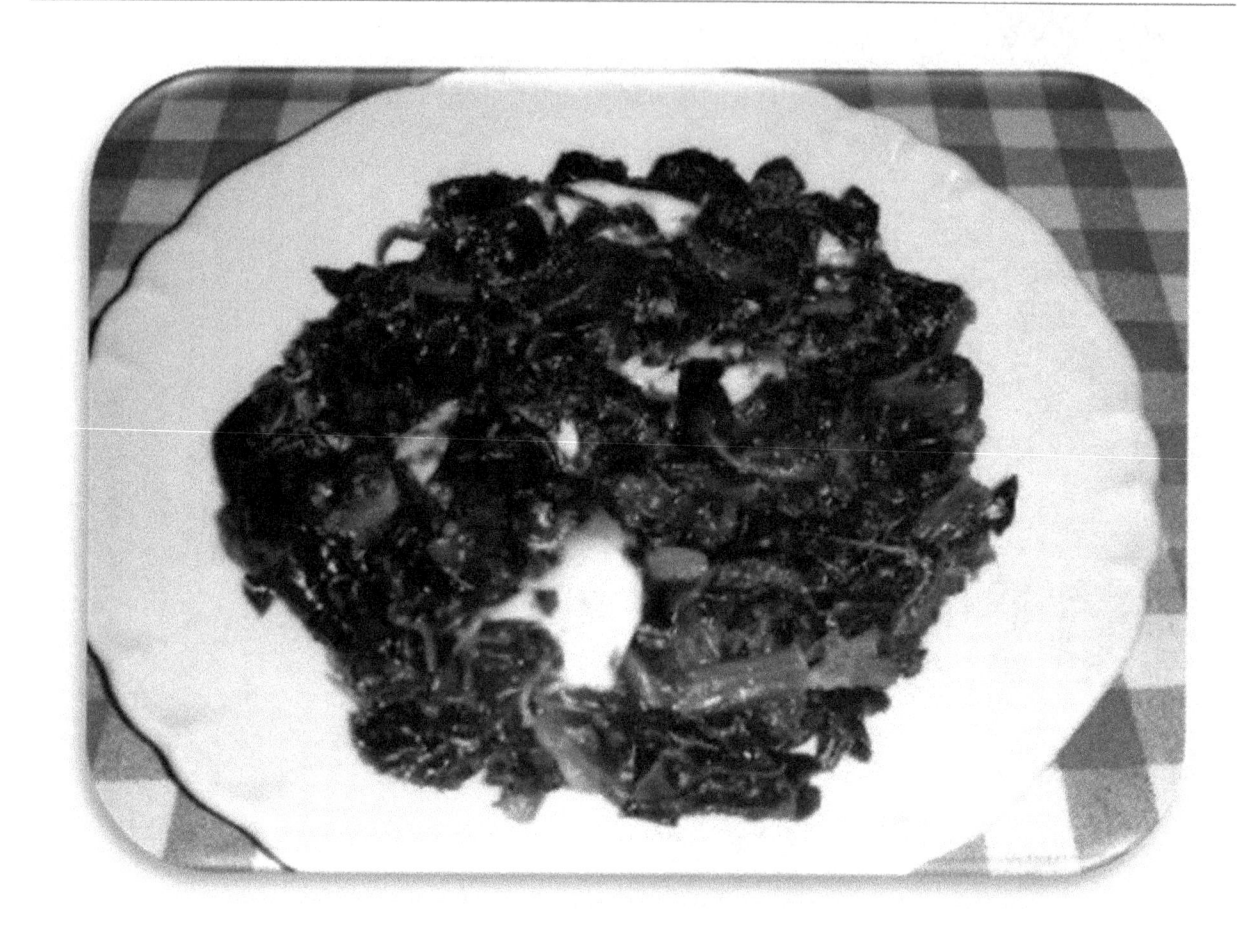

CARBS: 9 g | FAT: 14.7 g | PROTEIN: 13.3 g | CALORIES: 222

INGREDIENTS

- *2 cups fresh spinach leaves, rinsed*
- *1 cup Mozzarella, diced*
- *2 Tbsp olive oil*
- *1 Tbsp butter*
- *Salt and pepper to taste*

DIRECTIONS

1. Parboil the spinach leaves in boiling water for 4 minutes. Drain under cold water.
2. Heat olive oil and butter in a pan, add spinach leaves. Season with salt and pepper, and cook for 2 minutes.
3. Add Mozzarella to the pan and stir. Remove from the heat. Serve.

LETTUCE WRAPS

SERVINGS: 4 | PREP TIME: 5 min. | COOK TIME: 15 min.

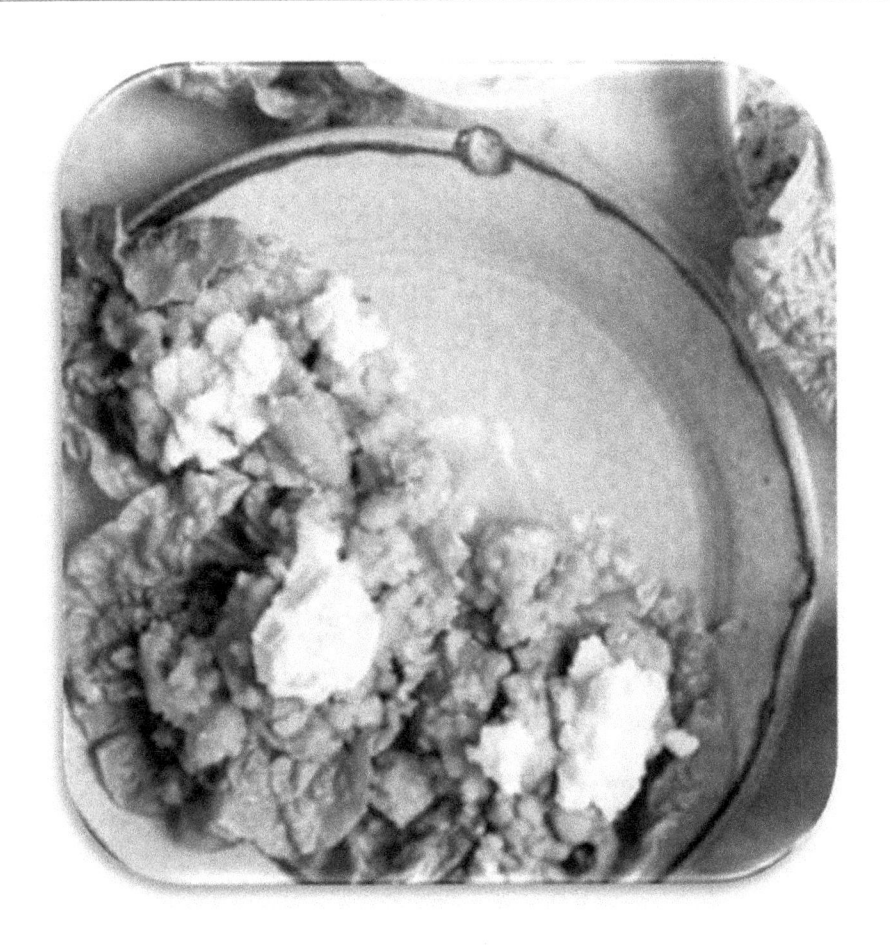

CARBS: 7.2 g | FAT: 36.4 g | PROTEIN: 50.9 g | CALORIES: 554

INGREDIENTS

- *1 chicken thigh, skinless, cut into 1 inch pieces*
- *7 lettuce leaves*
- *¼ cup onion, minced*
- *2 garlic cloves, minced*
- *1 cup cauliflower rice*
- *2 Tbsp butter*
- *½ cup sour cream*
- *2 tsp curry powder*
- *Salt and pepper to taste*

DIRECTIONS

1. Brown the onions in 2 Tbsp butter.
2. Add garlic and chicken, and season with salt.
3. Cook for about 8 minutes, stirring.
4. Add ¼ Tbsp butter, cauliflower rice and curry powder. Sauté until combined.
5. Spoon the chicken mix onto lettuce leaves.
6. Serve with sour cream.

BEVERAGES

LAVENDER GLASS

SERVINGS: 4 | PREP TIME: 1 h. 10 min. | COOK TIME: 5 min.

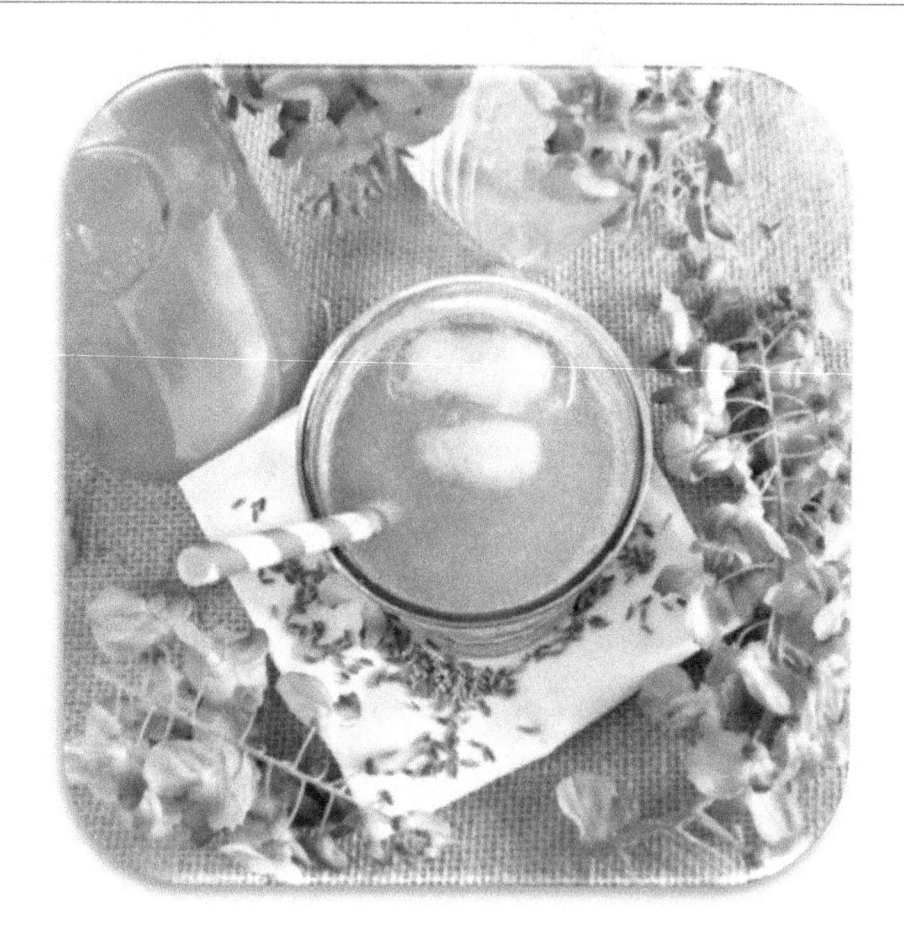

CARBS: 5.4 g | FAT: 0.3 g | PROTEIN: 0.6 g | CALORIES: 19

INGREDIENTS

- *2 Tbsp lavender flowers, dried*
- *3 lemons, juiced*
- *4½ cups water*
- *⅓ cup stevia extract, liquid*

DIRECTIONS

1. Add 2.5 cups of water to a skillet with lavender flowers and bring to boil. Reduce the heat and boil for 5 minutes. Remove from heat and let stand for 1 hour covered.
2. Filter the lavender flowers, add lemon juice and liquid stevia.
3. Pour the lemonade into a jar and place into the fridge to cool.

GINGER COOLER

SERVINGS: 1 cup | PREP TIME: 15 min. | COOK TIME: 2 min.

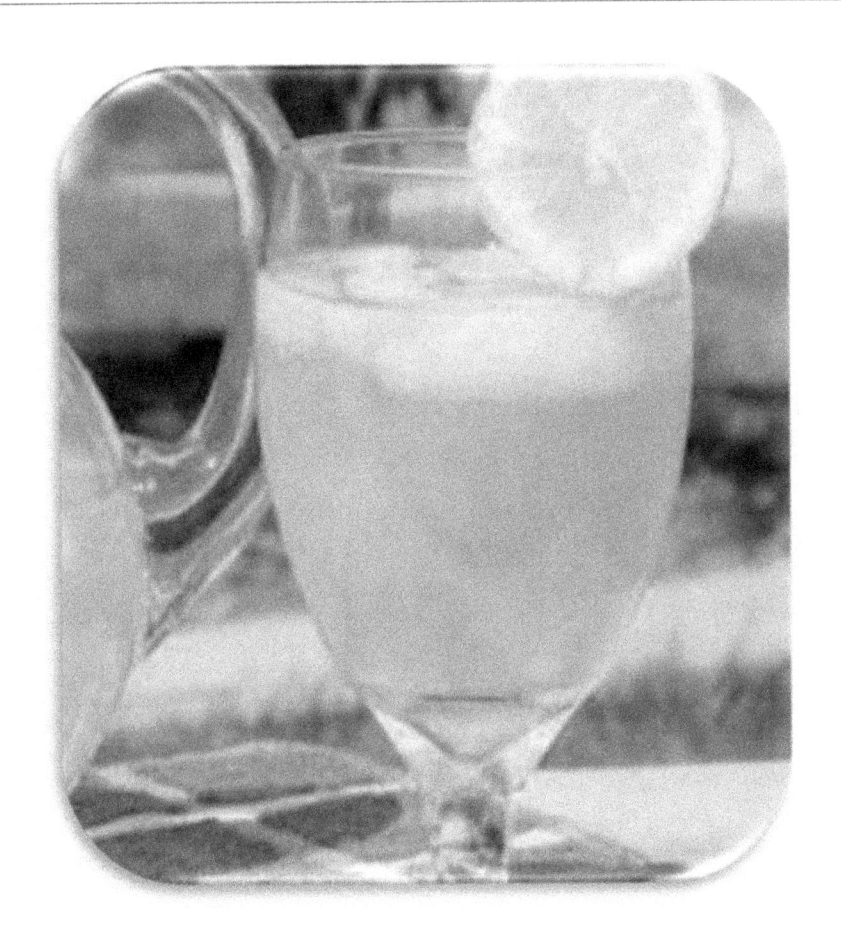

CARBS: 16 g | FAT: 2.1 g | PROTEIN: 2.3 g | CALORIES: 97

INGREDIENTS

- ½ cup water
- ½ cup lemon juice
- 2 inch piece ginger, peeled, sliced
- 1 tsp liquid stevia
- Sparkling water to serve
- Ice if desired

DIRECTIONS

1. Bring the water with stevia and ginger to a boil. Remove from heat and let cool.
2. Add the lemon juice.
3. Pour the syrup mixture through a sieve into a jar and store in the fridge.
4. To serve, mix some lemon-ginger syrup with sparkling water and ice.

APPLE PEEL TEA

SERVINGS: 2 | PREP TIME: 15 min. | COOK TIME: 15 min.

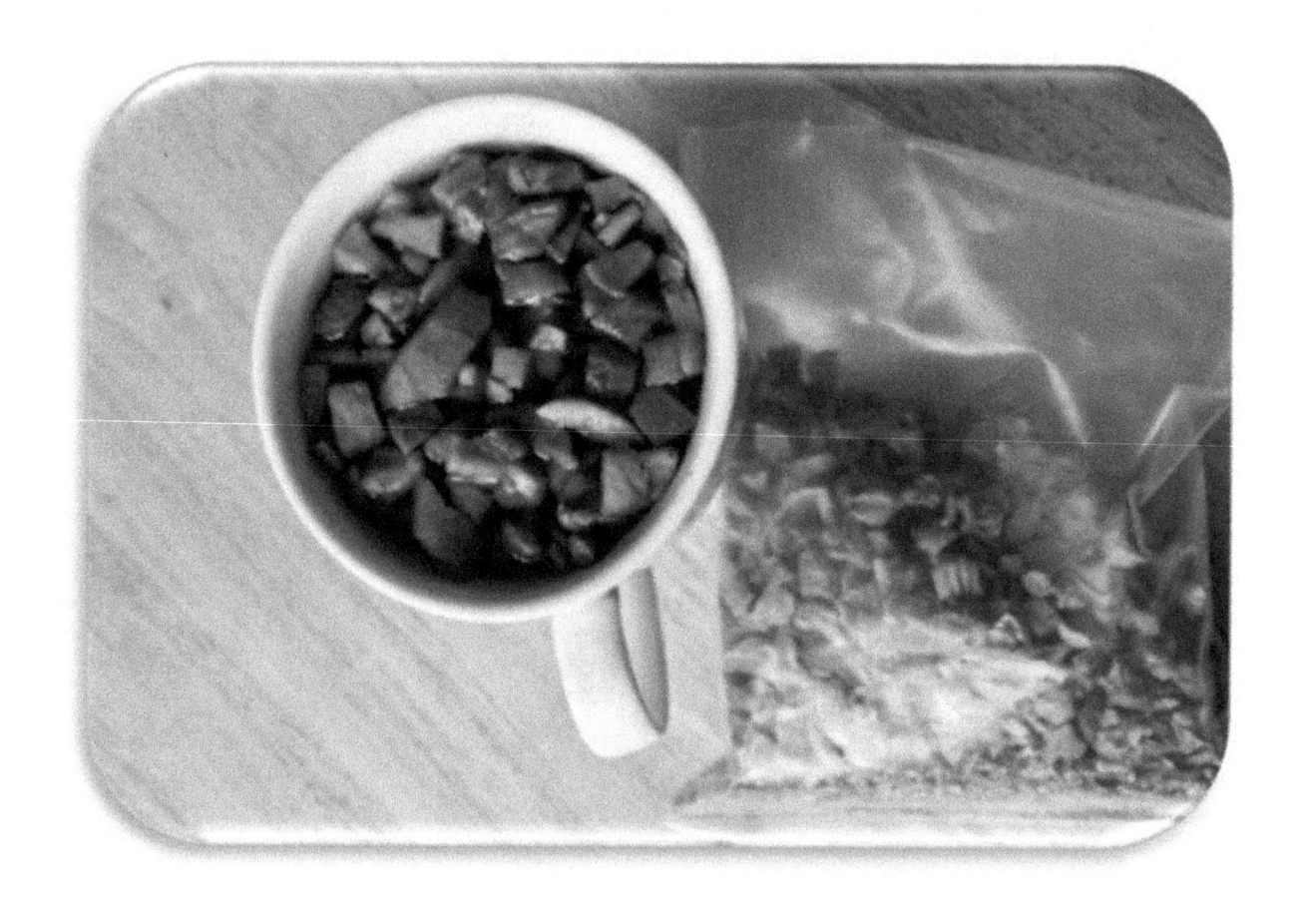

CARBS: 0.5 g | FAT: 0 g | PROTEIN: 0 g | CALORIES: 1

INGREDIENTS

- 3 Tbsp apple peel, dried
- 2 cups water
- ½ stick cinnamon
- Sweetener to taste

DIRECTIONS

1. Put dried apple peel and cinnamon into a pot.
2. Pour in water to cover and bring to a boil. Remove from the heat.
3. Let stand for 15 minutes, covered, and serve.

CILANRO BREW

SERVINGS: 1 | PREP TIME: 2 min. | COOK TIME: 15 min.

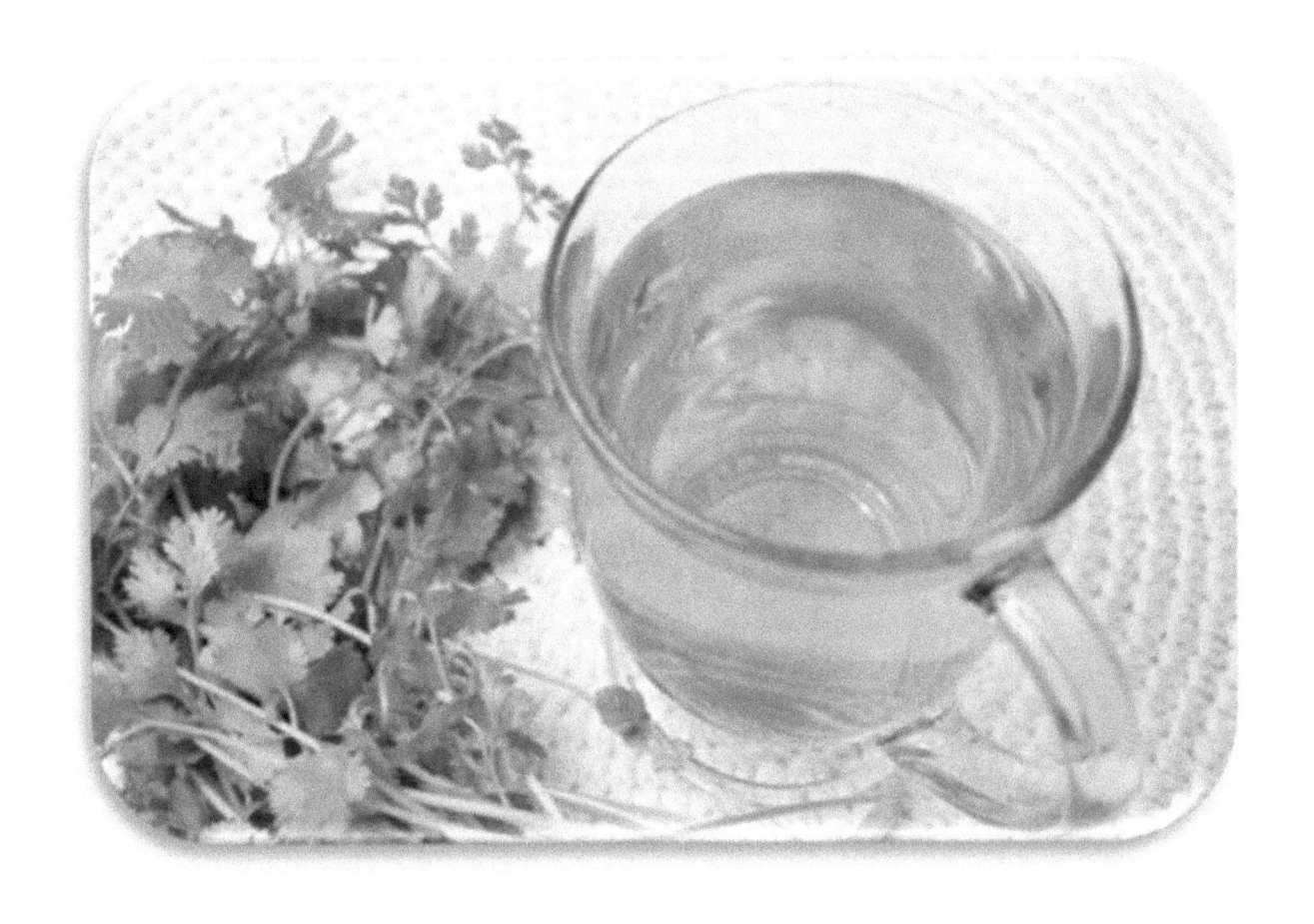

CARBS: 1 g | FAT: 00 g | PROTEIN: 0.5 g | CALORIES: 5

INGREDIENTS

- *1 Tbsp cilantro seeds or 2 Tbsp cilantro leaves*
- *1 cup boiling water*
- *Sweetener to taste*

DIRECTIONS

1. Pour boiling water over 1 Tbsp cilantro seeds or leaves and let stand, covered, for 15 minutes.
2. Add sweetener to taste and serve.

CHICORY COFFEE

SERVINGS: 2 | PREP TIME: 2 min. | COOK TIME: 12 min.

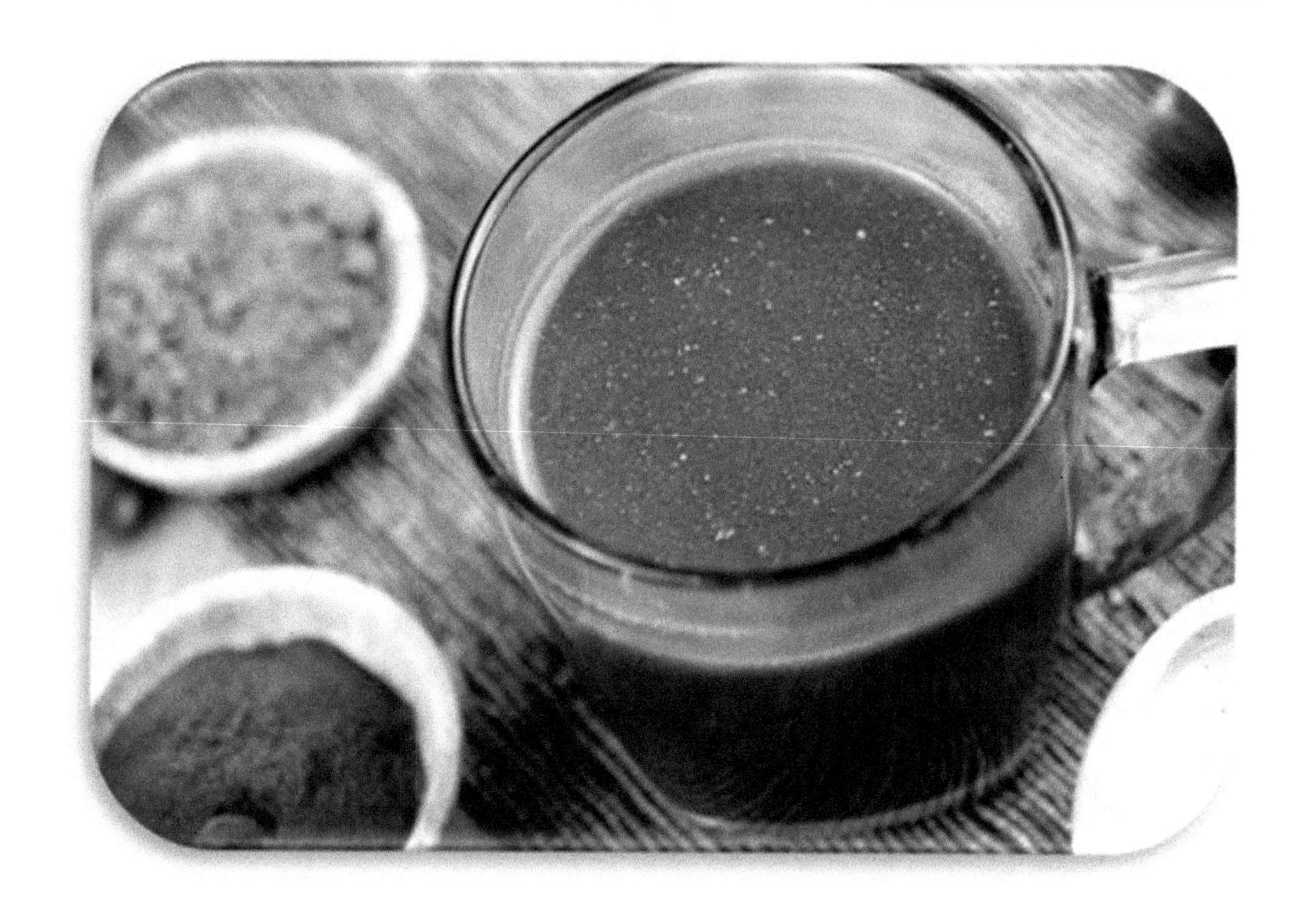

CARBS: 8 g | FAT: 18 g | PROTEIN: 2.1 g | CALORIES: 193

INGREDIENTS

- *2 Tbsp roasted chicory root*
- *2 Tbsp coconut butter*
- *Nutmeg to taste*
- *2 cups water*

DIRECTIONS

1. Place the chicory root into a pot and cover with water.
2. Bring to a boil and simmer for 2 minutes.
3. Remove from the heat and let stand for 5 minutes.
4. Strain into a bowl and transfer the liquid to a blender.
5. Blend with coconut butter and a dash of nutmeg.
6. Add sweetener to your coffee if desired and serve.

TURMERIC POWER

SERVINGS: 1 | PREP TIME: 1 min. | COOK TIME: 0 min.

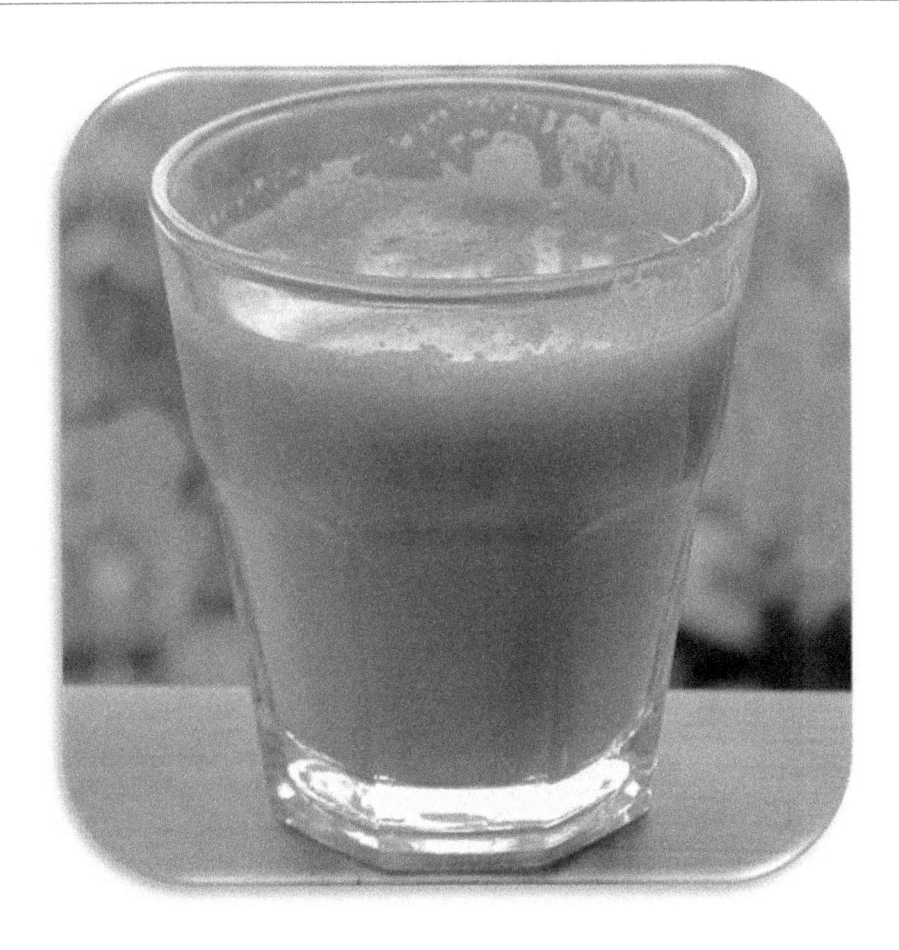

CARBS: 6 g | FAT: 10 g | PROTEIN: 1 g | CALORIES: 118

INGREDIENTS

- ½ cup whey
- 1 tsp turmeric powder
- ½ Tbsp flaxseed oil
- ½ cup water
- ½ cup tomato juice
- Dash of black pepper

DIRECTIONS

1. Combine all ingredients in a blender and pulse on high.
2. Serve.

COLD CHOCOLATE

SERVINGS: 3 | PREP TIME: 3 min. | COOK TIME: 0 min.

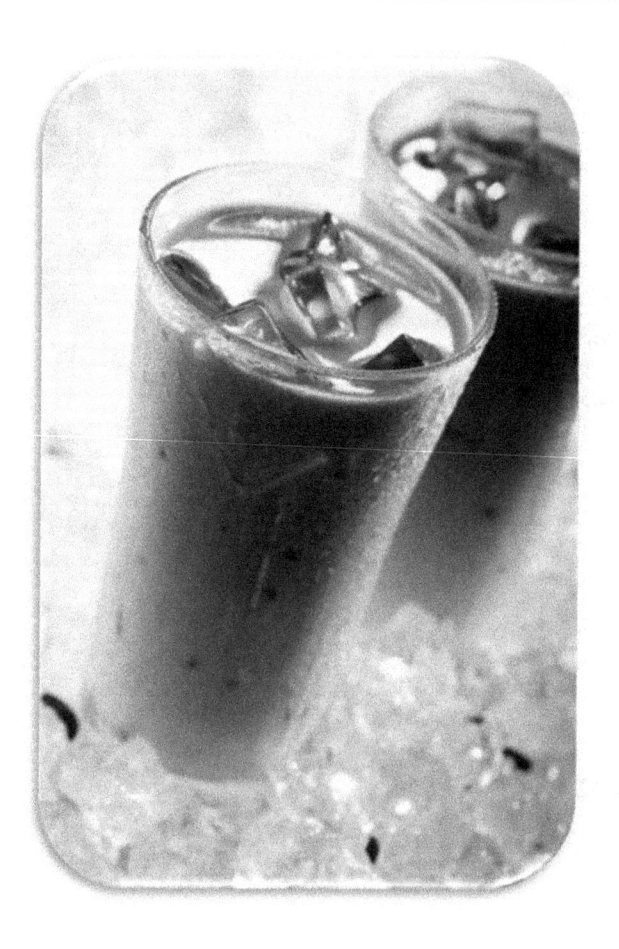

CARBS: 13.9 g | FAT: 7.7 g | PROTEIN: 5.7 g | CALORIES: 90

INGREDIENTS

- *1 cup freshly brewed coffee, cooled*
- *4 Tbsp cacao powder*
- *2 Tbsp coconut milk*
- *15 ice cubes, crushed in a blender*
- *Sweetener to taste (2-3 tsp)*

DIRECTIONS

1. Add all ingredients to a blender and pulse on high until smooth.
2. Serve.

VODKA MOJITO

SERVINGS: 1 | PREP TIME: 2 min. | COOK TIME: 0 min.

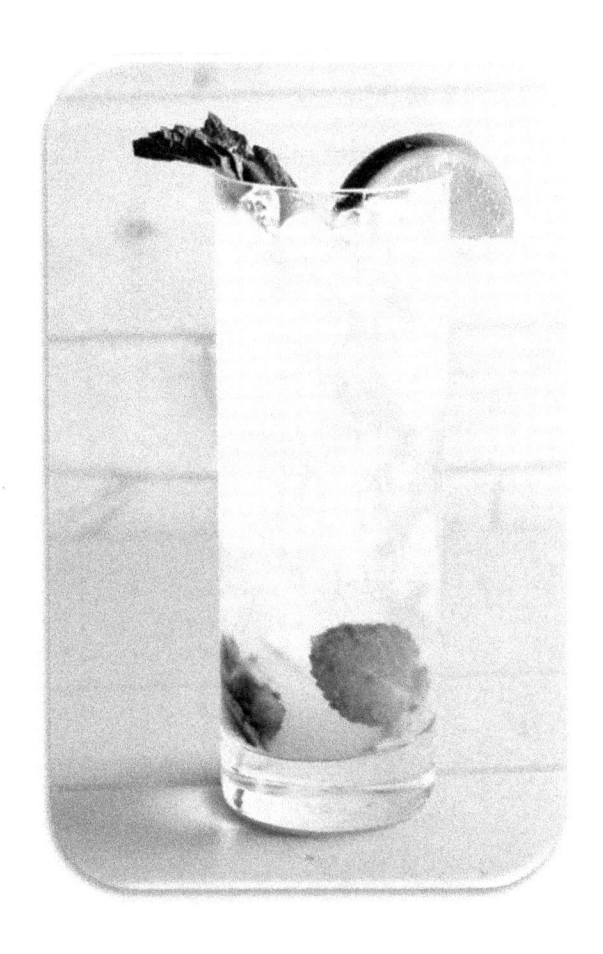

CARBS: 2 g | FAT: 0 g | PROTEIN: 0 g | CALORIES: 109

INGREDIENTS

- 1 shot vodka
- 1 splash club soda
- 2 Tbsp lime juice
- 2–3 tsp granulated stevia
- 4 fresh mint leaves (+more for garnish)
- Ice to taste

DIRECTIONS

1. Mash mint leaves with sweetener and lime juice in a glass.
2. Add ice to the glass.
3. Pour in vodka and soda. Garnish with mint leaves.

TOM COLLINS

SERVINGS: 1 | PREP TIME: 2 min. | COOK TIME: 0 min.

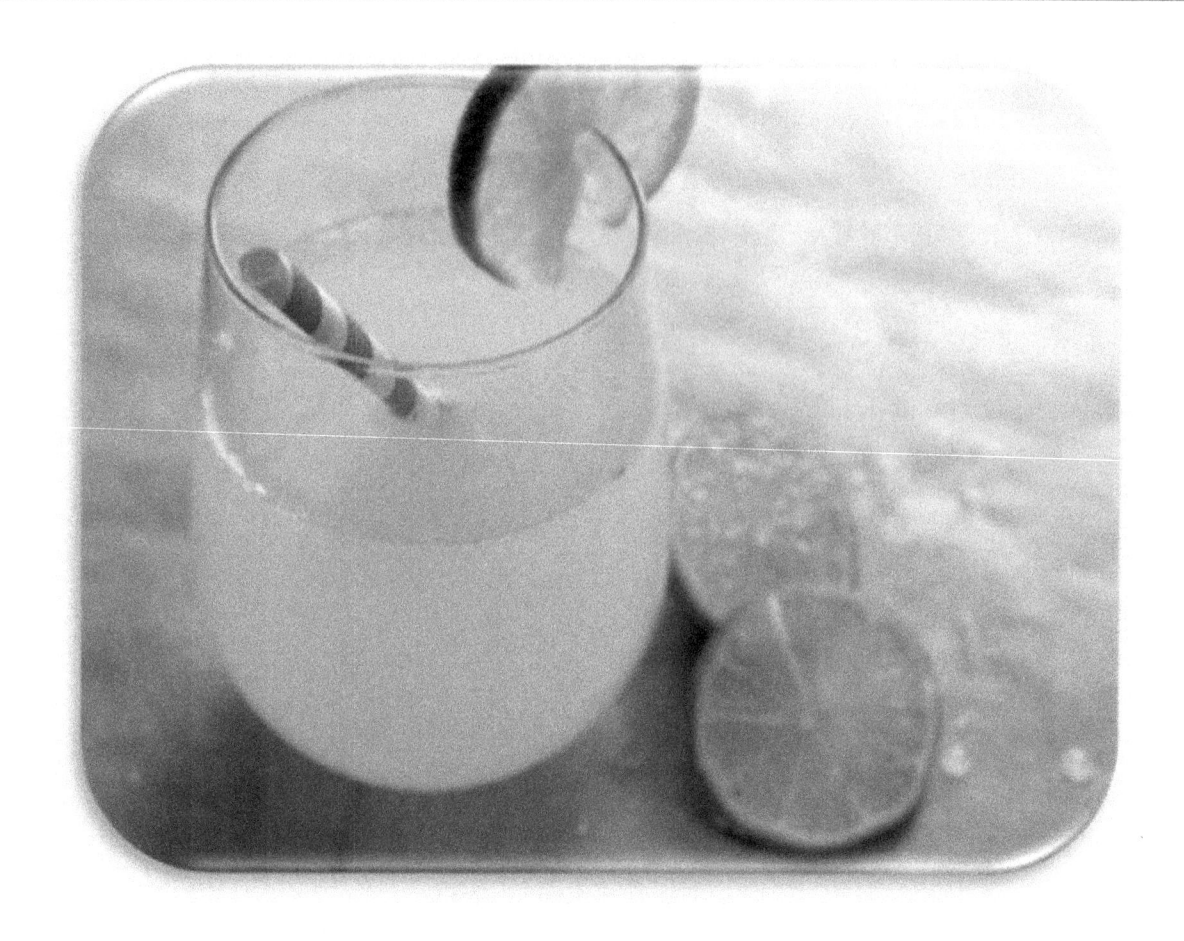

CARBS: 2 g | FAT: 0 g | PROTEIN: 9 g | CALORIES: 117

INGREDIENTS

- 3 oz gin
- Soda to taste (1-2 oz)
- 2 oz lemon juice
- 1 cup water
- 1 cup erythritol
- Lemon or lime slices
- 1 cup ice

DIRECTIONS

1. Prepare sweet syrup by bringing water with erythritol to a boil.
2. Cool the syrup.
3. Add gin, lemon juice, the syrup and 1 cup ice to a shaker.
4. Shake well and strain into a glass. Add soda.
5. Serve with lemon or lime slice.

WASABI MARGARITA

SERVINGS: 1 | PREP TIME: 1 min. | COOK TIME: 0 min.

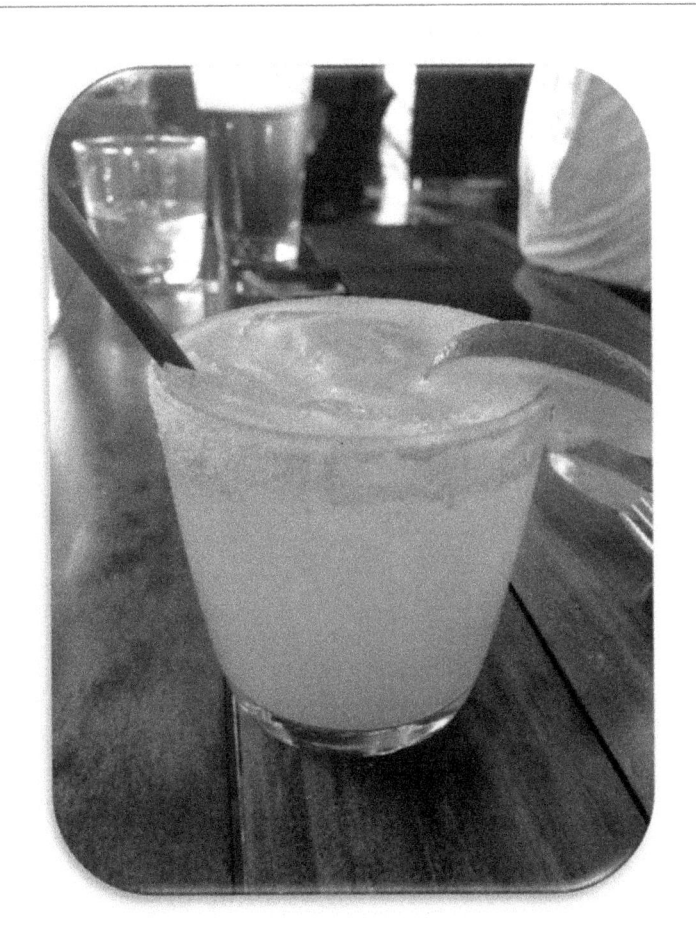

CARBS: 0.8 g | FAT: 0.5 g | PROTEIN: 0.2 g | CALORIES: 210

INGREDIENTS

- *1.6 oz tequila silver*
- *1.6 oz orange liqueur*
- *1 tsp wasabi*
- *1½ Tbsp lemon juice*
- *Ice to taste*

DIRECTIONS

1. Add orange liqueur, tequila, lemon juice, wasabi and ice to a shaker.
2. Shake well and transfer to a glass rimmed with salt.

CONCLUSION

Thank you for reading this book and having the patience to try the recipes.

I do hope that you have had as much enjoyment reading and experimenting with the meals as I have had writing the book.

If you would like to leave a comment, you can do so at the Order section–>Digital orders, in your account.

Stay safe and healthy!

RECIPE INDEX

A

Apple Peel Tea 65
Avocado and Ccumber Salad 39
Avocado and Shrimp Salad 38
Avocado and Tuna Brown Rice 48
Avocado Bars 50
Avocado Bowl 43
Avocado Casserole 44
Avocado Feta Dip 45
Avocado Ice Cream 49
Avocado Salad 41
Avocado Salsa 40
Avocado Sping Rolls 42

B

Bacon and Egg Fat Bombs 28
Bacon and Pear Salad 36
Bacon Salad with Walnuts 35
Bacon Ties 32
Bacon Wrapped Chicken 30
Bacon Wrapped Mozzarella 31
Broccoli and Mushroom Quiche 56
Broccoli in Orange Sauce 57
Broccoli Omelet 25

C

Cabbage and Egg Salad 52
Cabbage Patties 51
Chicken Fillets Baked with Broccoli
.... 55
Chicory Coffee 67
Cilantro Brew 66
Cold Chocolate 69
Cucumber Rolls with Avocado 47

E

Egg and Shrimp Salad 27
Egg Paste 23
Eggs Florentine 26

F

Fried Bacon and Cabbage 29

G

Ginger Cooler 64

Goat Cheese Frittata 19
Green Eastern Salad 54

K

Kale Salad 53

L

Laender Glass 63
Lettuce Wraps 62

M

Mediterranean Delived Eggs 22
Mozzarella Spinach 61
Mushrooms stuffed with Eggs 24

N

No Bread BLT 37

O

Omelet in a Cup 18

P

Prosciutto-Wrapped Avocado 46

R

Romaine Salad 33

S

Scotch Quali Eggs 21
Spinach Rolls 60
Spinach Salad with Tuna 59
Spinach with Tomatoes 58
Squash Frittata 20

T

Tom Collins 71
Turmeric Power 68

V

Vodka Mojito 70

W

Warm Bacon and Arugula Salad 34
Wasabi Margarita 72

CONVERSION TABLES

Dry Weights

OZ	Tbsp	C	g	lb
1/2 OZ	1 Tbsp	1/16 C	15 g	
1 OZ	2 Tbsp	1/8 C	28 g	
2 OZ	4 Tbsp	1/4 C	57 g	
3 OZ	6 Tbsp	1/3 C	85 g	
4 OZ	8 Tbsp	1/2 C	115 g	1/4 lb
8 OZ	16 Tbsp	1 C	227 g	1/2 lb
12 OZ	24 Tbsp	1 1/2 C	340 g	3/4 lb
16 OZ	32 Tbsp	2 C	455 g	1 lb

Liquid Conversions

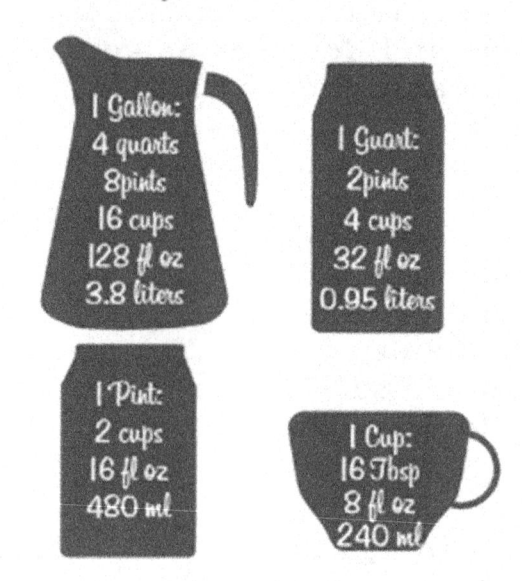

1 Gallon: 4 quarts, 8 pints, 16 cups, 128 fl oz, 3.8 liters

1 Quart: 2 pints, 4 cups, 32 fl oz, 0.95 liters

1 Pint: 2 cups, 16 fl oz, 480 ml

1 Cup: 16 Tbsp, 8 fl oz, 240 ml

Liquid Measures

OZ	tsp	Tbsp	mL	C	Pt	Qt
1 oz	6 tsp	2 Tbsp	30 ml	1/8 C		
2 oz	12 tsp	4 Tbsp	60 ml	1/4 C		
2 2/3 oz	16 tsp	5 Tbsp	80 ml	1/3 C		
4 oz	24 tsp	8 Tbsp	120 ml	1/2 C		
5 1/3 oz	32 tsp	11 Tbsp	160 ml	2/3 C		
6 oz	36 tsp	12 Tbsp	177 ml	3/4 C		
8 oz	48 tsp	16 Tbsp	237 ml	1 C	1/2 pt	1/4 qt
16 oz	96 tsp	32 Tbsp	480 ml	2 C	1 pt	1/2 qt
32 oz	192 tsp	64 Tbsp	950 ml	4 C	2 pt	1 qt

Fahrenheit to Celcius (F to C)

- 500 F = 260 C
- 475 F = 245 C
- 450 F = 235 C
- 425 F = 220 C
- 400 F = 205 C
- 375 F = 190 C
- 350 F = 180 C
- 325 F = 160 C
- 300 F = 150 C
- 275 F = 135 C
- 250 F = 120 C
- 225 F = 107 C

1 Tbsp: 15 ml
1 tsp: 5 ml

Safe Cooking Meat Temperatures

Minimum temperatures:

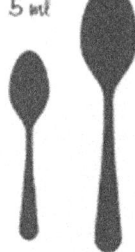

- **USDA Safe at 145 F:** Beef Steaks, Briskets, and Roasts; Pork Chops, Roasts, Ribs, Shoulders, and Butts; Lamb Chops, Legs, and Roasts; Fresh Hams, Veal Steaks, Fish, and Shrimp
- **USDA Safe at 160 F:** Ground Meats (except poultry)
- **USDA Safe at 165 F:** Chicken & Turkey, ground or whole

CPSIA information can be obtained
at www.ICGtesting.com
Printed in the USA
BVHW051503060221
599512BV00014B/2674